"*The Immunotherapy Revolution* is critical and essential reading for all cancer patients and their loved ones. More than recommend it—I insist on sharing it!"

— **Dr. Jeffrey Thompson**
founder of the Center for Neuroacoustic Research and
featured in documentary *Heal*

"Dr. Williams is a pioneer who, through courageous, tenacious pursuit, has identified a revolutionary approach to cancer that puts him at the cutting edge of what is possible in cancer healing."

—**Jim Roach**, MD, ABOIM, ABIHM
author of the highly acclaimed *Vital Strategies in Cancer*,
and Amazon #1 in 4 categories *God's House Calls.*

"I have had the opportunity and the pleasure to collaborate with Dr. Williams for many years. He is a wealth of knowledge and is always willing to push the envelope, in order to improve cancer treatments. I applaud his work and persistence in the arena of intra-tumoral immunotherapy. It is because of individuals like Dr. Williams, that there is still hope for a cure for this deadly disease. I highly encourage you to read *The Immunotherapy Revolution*."

— **Mark Rosenberg**, MD
founder of the Institute for Healthy Aging and
Integrative Cancer Therapeutics

"The work Dr. Jason Williams is doing is very powerful and truly healing people. He is really creating a revolution with his commitment, perseverance, and willingness to eradicate this disease. Do yourself a favor and read the *The Immunotherapy Revolution*."

— **Jack Canfield**
multiple New York Times bestselling author of the
Chicken Soup for the Soul® *series and The Power of Focus.*

THE
IMMUNOTHERAPY
REVOLUTION

THE IMMUNOTHERAPY REVOLUTION

THE BEST NEW HOPE FOR SAVING CANCER PATIENTS' LIVES

JASON R. WILLIAMS, MD, DABR

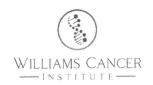

WILLIAMS CANCER INSTITUTE

Williams Cancer Institute
111 Myrtle Ave. Suite 1
Foley, Al 36535

ISBN: 9781700114938

This book is for my grandmother,

Effie Jenkins McIntyre,

whose fight against breast cancer left a lasting impression on this young boy.

In memory of my father, Jim, who passed away unexpectedly while I was in the middle of writing this book. He was one of the smartest people I have ever known. Dad, your belief in me always gave me comfort and motivation. Your advice, always wise. I wish you had been able to see the completion of this book; however, I made changes, just like you had recommended. I love you and miss you!

Contents

Foreword...xi

Introduction 1

Chapter 1: My Search For A Better Way To Treat Cancer 7

Chapter 2: What You Need to Know to Get Started:
The Basics of Cancer Immunotherapy...................................... 19

Chapter 3: Cancer and the Immune System............................. 33

Chapter 4: AblationVax™: The Cancer
Ablation "Vaccine" 39

Chapter 5: Intra-tumoral Immunotherapy
"The Cure is Within You"... 57

Chapter 6: Other Important Immunotherapy Targets
and Therapies 69

Chapter 7: The Effect of Traditional Cancer Treatments
On the Cancer Immune Response—The Good, The Bad
and The Ugly 75

Chapter 8: Genetic and Molecular Targeted Cancer
Drugs and Immunotherapy, Don't Miss Your Chance
For Synergy 85

Chapter 9: Gut Flora: The Key to Successful
Immunotherapy 95

Chapter 10: Unexpected Off-label Drugs To Boost
Your Immunity 113

Chapter 11: The Acidic Tumor Microenvironment
and Metabolic Immune Checkpoint 131

Chapter 12: Predicting Immunotherapy Response—
Laboratory Testing and Biomarkers 141

Chapter 13: Natural Substances and Supplements
to Enhance the Cancer Immune Response 147

Chapter 14: Immune Related Adverse Events and
Side Effects of Cancer Immunotherapy 157

Chapter 15: Dr. Williams's Cancer Immunotherapy
Pyramid and Plan to Maximize Success 169

Conclusion 173

Frequently Asked Questions 185
Resources 191
Acknowledgements 193
About the Author 197
Endnotes 199

Foreword

I HAVE KNOWN DR. Jason Williams for over a decade, have referred many patients to him, and have watched the development of his therapy over time and, indeed, participated to some extent in it with many discussions over the years.

I enthusiastically welcome his excellent book, which now brings information about his groundbreaking work to the public and to potentially interested physicians involved in cancer care.

Dr. Williams tells the story of the development of his pioneering work in an engaging way, yet liberally sprinkled with core science about immunotherapy and cancer and filled with key references for interested medical professionals to look up, as well as for patients and their families to print out and bring to their doctor.

He carries a high level of technical expertise with interventional radiology, developed through clinical experience in ablating malignant tumors in virtually every tissue of the body, which stretches back to the very beginning of his clinical education in radiology after completing medical school. He combines this interventional radiology expertise with a high level of knowledge about the science of immunology, cancer, and cancer immunotherapy.

As one of the founders of a new science of "Interventional Oncology," Jason is realistic about the challenges facing this nascent science.

The vast majority of people with cancer are treated by the three types of oncologists— surgical, medical, and radiation oncologists. As a medical oncologist myself, I was interested in immunotherapeutic approaches to treating cancer decades before the success of modern cancer immunotherapy literally burst on the scene with the approval of Yervoy (anti-CTLA-4 antibody) in 2011 plus Keytruda and Opdivo (anti-PD-1 antibodies) a few years later.

In his book, Dr. Williams describes the few dramatic examples of the 'abscopal effect', i.e. regression of other metastatic tumors not treated by thermal ablation, which happened only occasionally in his early years of work with "Interventional Oncology" but began to happen much more frequently after he was able to inject these sophisticated anti-cancer immuno-antibodies (the subject of the Nobel Prize in Medicine for 2018), into tumor deposits that he had just ablated by freezing or heating.

Injecting these antibodies directly into tumors (local treatment), rather than intravenously (systemic treatment), as they are conventionally given, appears to have dramatically increased the response rate and reduced the adverse side effects, as well as requiring much smaller quantities of these extremely expensive cancer medications (which can cost up to $30,000 per IV infusion).

On the face of it, there is a chance that the pharmaceutical industry might be unenthusiastic about a new therapy that uses far less of their product. However, it may also open the doors to successful treatment of a far broader spectrum of cancer patients than are currently benefited by the new immunotherapies. This would be a win for patients, doctors, and the pharmaceutical industry alike. In the beginning, it seems unlikely that the pharma industry will be interested in sponsoring clinical trials of this new therapeutic approach. Hopefully, government resources and philanthropic organizations will sponsor the large scale clinical trials needed to establish a practice changing therapy.

Another challenge Dr. Williams's new approach to cancer immunotherapy faces, as previously mentioned, is that neither surgical, radiation, nor medical oncologists are trained in the interventional radiology skills needed to thermally ablate tumor deposits and then inject 'cocktails' of immunotherapy agents directly into the ablated site, and they are not likely to want to turn over the treatment of their patients to interventional radiologists who do possess this skill set but don't have training in cancer biology nor management of cancer and its complications.

Dr. Williams sagely relates an analogous revolution that took place between the cardiology and cardiovascular surgical professions over the past few decades. In the mid 1960s, an interventional radiologist placed the first stent in a coronary artery of a patient with severe coronary disease. Prior to that seminal event, the dominant approach to coronary disease was coronary artery bypass grafting, done exclusively by cardiovascular surgeons. However, once the cardiology profession began to train young cardiologists in the interventional radiology procedures necessary to place stents into blocked or nearly blocked coronary arteries, the modern science of 'interventional cardiology' was born, and cardiologists became able to have a much larger role in the treatment of severe coronary artery disease, although surgical management is still used in certain situations.

A similar transformation is possible within either (or all) the professions of medical, radiation, and surgical oncology. If young doctors are trained in the interventional techniques necessary to ablate tumor deposits by freezing or heating and subsequently inject immunotherapy agents directly into ablated tumor sites, the stage will be set for the pioneering work of Dr. Williams to become widely accepted and practiced, should randomized clinical trials of this approach prove it to be superior to current immuno-oncology approaches, as I believe will prove to be the case.

Dr. Williams covers the critical areas not only of the innovative use of natural products and 'off-label' drugs (drugs not conventionally used in oncology) to support cancer immunotherapy but also the crucial roles that diet, lifestyle, and stress management play in fueling and maintaining an effective immune response against cancer.

I urge all readers to enjoy this exciting glimpse into the future, and begin to apply it now.

— Dwight L. McKee, MD, CNS, ABIHM
author of *After Cancer Care*

Introduction

I F YOU'VE PICKED up this book, it is probably because you or someone you know and love has cancer. You're hoping to learn something about the exciting breakthroughs in immunotherapy treatment. I have written this book to help you understand exactly what the treatment is, what it entails, and what you can do to improve the chances the treatment will be effective.

Cancer is not a new disease. Fossilized tumors have been found in the bones of mummies dating as far back as 3,000 B.C. To the best of our knowledge, cancer was not as common back then as it is today. Perhaps this was because people lived much shorter lives back then, or maybe the increasing prevalence of cancer today is related to more toxic exposures and diet in our current modern life. Now, it is estimated that nearly 40% of the nation will receive a cancer diagnosis in their lifetime.[1] Cancer is now the second leading cause of death in the United States, with an estimated 1.7 million new cases diagnosed each year. That's grim news and it means that cancer has affected, or will soon affect, virtually everyone in some way.

To be diagnosed with cancer is devastating, not only because of the nature of the disease itself, but also because conventional treatments can be excruciating, debilitating, and may not even work. The typical treatment for cancer has pretty much amounted to cut, poison and burn. Through surgery, toxic chemotherapy, and radiation, our aggressive efforts to eliminate any traces of cancer have left patients with bodies often as ravaged by the treatment as the disease itself.

But there's good news. Recent scientific advancements in the diagnosis and treatment of cancer have led to amazing breakthroughs in our understanding of how to treat it, and in many cases, eliminate any trace of cancer cells. And one of the most remarkable of these advancements has been in immunotherapy. Immunotherapy became widely known when former President Jimmy Carter's medical team used it to treat his cancer. When the former president announced in August, 2015 that malignant tumors had been found in both his liver and his brain, most people presumed that he would be dead within months. But just four months later he surprised the world with the news that, following a remarkable and revolutionary new treatment, there was no sign of cancer in his body. The treatment he received was a drug classified as an "immune checkpoint inhibitor". This class of medications has kicked off a revolution that has demonstrated that cancer can be cured by your own immune system. It just needs a little help. There are now countless drugs based on this principle. What these are and how to maximize your chances in the fight against cancer is the focus of this book.

In the chapters that follow you will learn:

- How and why optimizing your body's immune system offers the best hope for preventing and treating cancer.

- How the immune system is designed to work to target and eliminate cancer before it takes hold in the body, and what can cause the immune system to become compromised, thwarting this process.

- The exciting promise of ablation therapy and how it acts like a potent cancer "vaccine".

- How and why intra-tumoral immunotherapy is proving that the cure for cancer is already within you.

- Other important immunotherapy targets and therapies that you need to know about.

- The "good, bad, and ugly" effects of traditional cancer treatments on the cancer immune response.

- The synergistic benefits of genetic and molecular targeted cancer drugs combined with immunotherapy.

I've also included chapters on the gut flora and why it is another key factor for successful immunotherapy outcomes, the surprising synergistic effect of aspirin and off-label drugs that can further boost immunity, beneficial nutritional supplements and other natural substances that may also be helpful, and other things that the patient can do to make the difference between success and failure. Many of these recommendations are not well known and most oncologists will probably not know to tell you about them. That is why it is up to you to play an active role in your care to ensure you have the best likelihood of success. These are things that patients getting standard FDA-approved systemic immunotherapy can benefit from as well.

In addition, I will discuss the new advances in intra-tumoral immunotherapy, which is the most advanced and successful delivery method of immunotherapy. This technique involves injecting cancer drugs right into the tumor. It's holding great potential for reducing side effects and ultimately to reduce the cost of treatment. Most importantly, it allows for a unique combination of medications that could not be used systemically (IV or oral) while also obtaining far superior results.

Keeping with the theme of intra-tumoral immunotherapy, you will also learn about the combination of OX40 and TLR agonist that was published by Dr. Levy in the *Stanford Cancer Vaccine* study. This study made major news as a potential cure for cancer because the treatment cured all the mice that received it.

I know what you are thinking: They cure mice all the time, when are they going to treat humans? We know that a cure in mice does not always translate into humans. I agree, treating actual people is more complicated, but in this study they were able to cure some difficult cancers, so this holds more promise than a typical mouse study. Which is why this is the same type of treatments I am doing already with humans. My work with patients looks promising as well, though realistically, I would not expect it to equal the results in mice. Yet even if it only works half as well, it would be the best cancer treatment ever discovered.

In the chapter on gut flora we will discuss which bacteria are essential components for the function of immunotherapy and you will learn that most typical probiotics either do not contain these bacteria or not enough of them to be significantly beneficial.

In the chapter on aspirin, I will explain how simple aspirin therapy can increase the effectiveness of immunotherapy. I will tell you about how a prescription medication for diabetes increased the effectiveness of immunotherapy in animals, and may do it in humans as well. And I will also discuss how adding immunotherapy to treatments like image-guided radiofrequency, microwave and cryoablation can create an effective tumor vaccine, significantly improving the results of any of these treatments alone.

My hope in writing this book is to provide you with clear and concise information that will enable you to take an active role in your cancer treatment. My goal is for cancer patients and their families to learn what can be added to standard therapies which may significantly improve their outcomes. I hope you will find this book helpful in enhancing your cancer treatment and will lead you to the road of a possible cure. We now have that cure for cancer within our sights, and while there is still more to go before this deadly disease is fully eradicated, we have reached the beginning of the end. And that end begins right here, with this book you hold in your hands.

CHAPTER 1

My Search For A Better
Way To Treat Cancer

EVER SINCE I was a young boy, I've been passionate about seeking the best solutions for helping others beat cancer. My passion was kindled because of one person— my beloved grandmother. It is because of her that I became interested in oncology—the study of cancer—which led me to become one of the leading practitioners of the amazing, minimally invasive image-guided technique that delivers maximum benefits of immunotherapy directly into tumors that this book is about.

When I was ten years old, my grandmother was diagnosed with breast cancer. The news was devastating. I was close to her, and during her sickness I became even closer, visiting her several times a week. She worked at the local high school, in the cafeteria. She was a very good cook, and we spent hours talking about food and how to prepare it. Those talks not only sparked my love of cooking, but of science, because she was always coming up with new ideas and discussing the science behind how to create the most flavorful foods, whether it was how to roast a chicken perfectly, make a perfect pie crust or whip up a stiff meringue. But perhaps my most memorable times with my grandmother were on Sundays when she'd make spaghetti with the best sauce I'd ever tasted—along with one giant meatball. I sure miss those meals.

Over the next two years, she grew progressively ill and by the time I was twelve she passed away, and along with her passing, I lost those wonderful meals and conversations. But I gained an insight into patient care and illness that have stayed with me to this day. Having watched how badly she suffered during her final years as she endured chemotherapy, surgery and radiation, I thought there had to be a better way to treat such a terrible disease. Maybe there was something right under our noses, I thought, something that we weren't noticing. Something that would be more effective and less tortuous than the agony of cutting off body parts, poisoning the patient, and burning them from the inside out. I was only a child, but I knew there had to be a better way and I would do my best to help find it.

When I started college majoring in chemistry, I became interested in gene therapy. I was fortunate to be able to enter a summer research program for gene therapy used in cancer treatment, a joint project of Tulane University, Louisiana State University and Ochsner Hospital in New Orleans. While working under the direction of some of the most gifted scientists in the field, I became enthusiastic about the future of gene therapy as a first-course treatment in cancer. The potential for gene therapy to radically alter how we treat the disease was nearly limitless, but two things about it really stood out. The first was that, although there was a long way to go in research, the potential for gene therapy to enhance the immune response against cancer was significant. The second was that in order for gene therapy to work, it probably had to be delivered directly into the tumor itself. Tucking those two ideas in the back of my mind, I returned to school that fall excited about my future career in medicine.

When I entered medical school at Louisiana State University in 1996, I was determined to be an oncologist. But by the end of my first year I attended a lecture that would change that plan and set me off in the direction of image-guided procedures. The lecture was on the topic of "Interventional Radiology", which is a minimally invasive way to use CT scans, ultrasound, and X-rays to help physicians treat a variety of health problems. Up until that point, I thought of radiologists as being limited to making a diagnosis, but not necessarily treating patients. Interventional radiology was somewhat unknown at the time, but was rapidly growing. Imaging techniques normally used to make a diagnosis can also help physicians to expertly guide needles or catheters through the body to reach organs or arteries without having to cut open the body. By using interventional radiology, the doctor can literally see inside the body, thereby delivering life-saving technologies and medicines with minimal risk to the patient.

The physician who was lecturing us on this topic was discussing the many ways that interventional radiology is used in clinical and surgical settings. At one point in the lecture he showed how it was used to perform image-guided biopsies of cancer at almost every location in the body—without surgery. At that moment, my memories of what I'd learned about gene therapy a few summers earlier came back to me, and I realized that the future of cancer treatment would not be limited to delivering medicines by mouth or through an IV. The future of cancer treatment would focus on injecting these medicines—and other technologies—directly into tumors—through imaging, not surgery.

I started spending as much free time as possible hanging out in radiology labs and reading up on the latest advancements in radiology—a field that was taking off as the technology was rapidly changing. I absorbed all the information on interventional radiology as fast as I could read it, attended every lecture on the topic that I could, and discussed my interest with every professor who would take the time to listen. Then one day a professor suggested that I contact one of his former radiology residency graduates working on image-guided ablation of cancer.

Ablation, precisely defined, is destroying something. The term is used more broadly to refer to freezing or destruction by heat, right inside the body. I learned that my professor's former medical resident, now a professor, was inserting needles into tumors using imaging, and then killing the tumor by directly freezing it—a process known as cryoablation—or heating it up with radio frequencies.

This was the most exciting thing I had heard in all my medical training. I imagined my grandmother having been spared the mastectomy that disfigured her, the poisons that had so debilitated her, the loss of her hair and body functions that had so humiliated her. Even if she hadn't ultimately been cured, if there had been a less invasive, more precise way to target the tumors in her breasts, she could have enjoyed her final years in much less pain.

I contacted the physician who was teaching and practicing at the University of Mississippi and arranged to spend the summer in an externship program where I could observe him in practice and learn as much as possible about his remarkable treatment. That summer was an eye-opener for me, and my own future in immunotherapy and cryoablation was set. I graduated from medical school and entered my residency in radiology at the University of South Alabama and shared my enthusiasm with our professor of interventional radiology. I explained that I wanted to apply ablation techniques to cancer treatment using interventional radiology, and he told me that if I could set it up, we could do it. I began contacting medical equipment companies to get the necessary equipment, and writing articles on the topic. I started a website and soon we had patients. I even contacted news outlets and it wasn't long before we had more patients than we could handle. With all of these, the future specialty of Interventional Oncology was born.

One of those patients was the mother of a medical colleague who had been treated for breast cancer. Her cancer had spread and she had developed lung metastasis. When we examined her, we found that she had four lung lesions—two in each lung. At that point in time we only considered ablation when the disease was limited—and mostly only in the liver because it was the easiest to treat through our method. But our colleague pleaded with us to make an attempt, because, with the tumors spreading to the lungs, it was clear her mother would die soon if something wasn't done. So we decided to give it a shot.

I felt that treating both lungs at the same time would add a lot of risk. But if we broke it up into two procedures, treating one lung first and then another several weeks later, we stood a better chance of the patient not running into extra complications. So we went ahead with the first procedure, using computed tomography (CT). Computed tomography is an imaging procedure using special X-ray equipment that allows us to see detailed images of the body's organs similar to what would be seen if you were able to cut right into them. Using CT, we guided our needles directly to the tumors and used radiofrequency ablation to heat up the tumors and destroy them. The procedure worked. Those two tumors had not only been killed; they were completely gone.

A few weeks later, our patient returned for the second procedure. We had her prepped for surgery and did the scan to determine exactly where the tumors were. And what we saw astounded us. Or better yet, what we didn't see astounded us. The other two tumors had also disappeared! We had done nothing to them, and she was not receiving any chemotherapy or other treatments to explain the disappearance of the tumors. But they had disappeared. It was at that moment that I realized that the ablation had stimulated her immune system, essentially acting like a vaccine of sorts. When I thought about it, this made sense. Vaccines are made from weakened or killed forms of disease microbes that are injected into the body. Once they are injected, the body's immune system then develops antibodies to attack the microbes, thinking they're a danger. We had killed the first two tumors using ablation. Perhaps in the process we had stimulated the body's immune response to attack the other tumors.

We had helped our patient, and made an astounding and intriguing scientific discovery. We still had a long way to go, but I was on my way to what would become a seventeen-year journey to determine how to make that successful outcome the norm and not the exception.

There was not much data at that time on how ablation could stimulate an anti-cancer immune response, and, as I was to find, that one case was not a common occurrence. But the fact that it had happened was enough for me to know that it could happen again once we had a better understanding of the process. I began researching ablation and tumors and found literature dating as far back as the 1960's where other procedures using crude ablation techniques (such as putting liquid nitrogen directly on tumors) had resulted in a complete immune response. The possibilities were clear. We just needed the right drug, or combination of drugs, to inject into the ablated tumor to make it happen.

As my work in the area of immunotherapy and ablation continued, however, I was to discover that the road to success could often become the road to ruin. Insurance companies would not cover the ablation procedures and it wasn't long before the university put a stop to our work in that area because they weren't being compensated. Fortunately, the Chairman and Residency Program Director of my department recognized the importance of my work and supported me in my efforts to continue. After I arranged to use facilities outside the university, he told me that if I wanted to take a leave from my residency and focus on the procedure, I could do so. He gave me two years before I had to return to finish up my residency and I accepted. I spent the next two years focusing exclusively on ablation.

During that time, I had other patients with advanced stage cancer who showed complete responses after being treated with ablation, including more tumors disappearing that had not been directly ablated. Of those with advanced disease who ultimately did not survive, I still noticed they did much better and lived longer than expected. I was convinced that the immune response had something to do with it.

By 2005, I began exploring what agents could be injected into tumors that could enhance more positive responses and result in more cures. The immunotherapy agents available at that time were extremely limited, mostly just Interleukin 2 and Interferon. It was also at this time that I learned that another researcher in the Netherlands, Martijn Den Brok, was also pursuing the same research. He had published several animal studies showing that ablation does cause an anti-cancer immune response. Den Brok[2] was also interested in CTLA-4, which plays a critical role in cancer production. CTLA-4 is a protein receptor that suppresses the immune response. Den Brok was studying the experimental immune checkpoint inhibitor, anti-CTLA-4. The current anti-CTLA-4 drug is more commonly known as Ipilimumab, or Yervoy—a medication that would later be approved by the Food and Drug Administration (FDA) in 2011. It was this drug that really started everything moving in the immunotherapy front, though it would mostly take a backseat to the more popular PD-1 inhibitors such as Keytruda and Opdivo, which would get approval a few years later. This is not to diminish the value of CTLA-4 inhibitors. They are just as important, maybe more so, in the right setting.

Den Brok also used studies from mice to show how the vaccine adjuvant, Matrix M or Saponin, enhanced the immune response of ablation. This finding was significant and energized my pursuit to explore cancer and the immune response.

I applied to the company making Matrix M so that we could try it ourselves. Although it had not yet been approved by the FDA, this agent was well studied and close to approval as a vaccine adjuvant, so we got a waiver which allowed us to use it. The technique of combining Matrix M with ablation had never been tried before in humans, so the patients that I was treating would become the first to undergo this procedure.

Starting with three patients, we combined ablation with Matrix M injected directly into their tumors. The first patient, MC (patients are not named so as to protect their privacy), had a non-small cell lung cancer. After a couple of ablation treatments in combination with Matrix M her tumors disappeared. Eight years later, as of this writing, she is still alive and well without any recurrence of her cancer.

The second patient, SM, was more challenging. He was 80 years old and had Stage IV renal (kidney) cancer. He had numerous tumors in his lungs and his kidney, which had the original cancer, removed. He had failed all the latest and greatest treatments for kidney cancer we had at that time.

Because he was older and had numerous health issues, we decided we could not be as aggressive with ablation as we would have liked. Consequently, we performed a cryoablation of one lesion and injected Matrix M into the tumor. Over the next few months, we were amazed to see that all but one of his tumors disappeared. That one tumor never really grew, however, remaining about one centimeter in size until he died six years later. And when he did die, it was not from cancer, but from an infection that he acquired following an injury to his leg from a fall. Although he had been given less than six months to live at the age of 81, following the ablation and Matrix M injection, he had lived to be 87 and was spared the long and devastating death that cancer so often brings.

The third patient we worked with that year, GM, was 32 years old and had Stage IV colon cancer, which had advanced throughout his body. There were tumors in his lungs and throughout most of his liver. Although we performed the ablation with Matrix M and the initial results were good, the cancer did come back. He lived a few more years, which was longer than expected, but died at the age of 35, right when we were making our real advance with immune checkpoint inhibitors in late 2014.

These three cases had demonstrated that we were on the right path, and encouraged me to continue my exploration in this area. There were rough years and at times I found myself discouraged as I continued to battle many obstacles, but I knew I couldn't give up. I took a private practice job, which kept me busy and limited the time I could devote to ablation, but it allowed me to have more money to put into my research.

As I spent the next few years looking at different agents and combinations of agents, the road certainly didn't get any easier. I had dedicated my entire life to this quest, and my personal and family life suffered for it. And I suffered, as well. My father pleaded with me to just be a regular doctor, telling me he didn't want me to end up like so many other scientists who had made great discoveries. Reminding me of the story of Nikola Tesla, probably one of the greatest scientists in history, my father pointed out that despite his contribution to science, Tesla had lived a very sad life and was never fully appreciated, at least not while he was alive. But I was driven; there was no way that I could stop. So like sons so often do, I did not listen to my father's advice to be a regular doctor, and continued my research in immunotherapy and cancer, and doing everything possible to help my patients defy the odds and eradicate their tumors. I'm happy and grateful to report that my persistence and ongoing research has paid off.

Since those early years, I have treated thousands of patients with advanced stage cancer and had remarkable results, including numerous complete remissions and cures. There have been more struggles than I can detail, but it has all been worth it, and I think very soon, these treatments that I now specialize in will become the standard for cancer therapies.

As you will learn in the pages that follow, immunotherapy is rapidly reaching the mainstream as a viable cancer treatment—in part due to Jimmy Carter's remarkable remission. Combining immunotherapy with cryoablation or direct injection of these medications into the tumor is even more promising. Read on to find out why.

In the pages that follow I will first discuss some basic principles of immunotherapy so that you'll have a better understanding of what the treatment is, how it works, and what it entails for the patient. As you read, you may come across medical and scientific terms that confuse you. If so, don't despair. I've done my best to explain what each is and highlight the important aspects that can enhance cancer treatment. I purposely did not want to make it into a science research book, but more of a guide for the patient. I have included the information needed to do further research. I strongly suggest that any patient do their own research, since no one has more at stake than you. As with any outside recommendations, you should always also discuss these with your doctor. But the final decision needs to be made by you. In the chapters that follow you will learn all that you need to know to decide wisely.

CHAPTER 2

What You Need to Know to Get Started: The Basics of Cancer Immunotherapy

C UT, POISON AND burn. Until recently, those have pretty much been the only choices cancer patients have had to treat their disease. They could cut out their tumors—and often a few body parts; poison their bloodstreams with chemical cocktails, and burn their bodies with radiation, which itself can cause other cancers. But in the past few years there has been a paradigm shift in cancer treatment, from medications that poison cancer to new medicines that unlock the body's own ability to destroy cancer through the immune system.

The concept of using the immune system to treat cancer is not new. In fact, it dates to the late nineteenth century when Dr. William Coley observed that patients who developed bacterial infections following cancer surgery sometimes fared better than non-infected patients. Hypothesizing that the infected incisions caused the immune system to become active, Coley tried to explore this line of treatment by deliberately infecting patients with bacteria. Certainly in the time before antibiotics, this created some problems, but it also resulted in some surprising successes as well. Unfortunately, his efforts were soon overshadowed by the development of radiation and chemotherapy. Sometimes the best does not always win out, just recall the video format wars between VHS and Betamax. Betamax had superior picture and sound quality, but VHS won out and dominated the market until the rise of DVD.

While Dr. Coley was initially optimistic about the potential for radiation to burn away tumors, the primitive state of X-ray technology led him to eventually determine it was ill suited as an effective cancer treatment. While others disagreed, and continued working in radiation treatment, Coley continued to study the effects of the immune system on cancer. In the meantime, chemotherapy became the mainstay of cancer therapy, despite its overall poor record of success. Even though Dr. Coley's work was for the most part ignored during his lifetime, today he is recognized as the "Father of Immunotherapy" for his contributions to this now burgeoning medical science.

Following Dr. Coley's death in 1936, radiation, chemo-therapy and surgery remained the standard cancer treatment for the next half-century and immunotherapy was relegated to the back burners of scientific research.

By the 1980's, however, scientists began to reconsider the idea of using the immune response to treat cancer. Though the scientific understanding of the immune system was much better than it had been in Dr. Coley's day, the results of these early efforts were disappointing. It seemed that no matter what technique was used to stimulate the immune system to attack cancer, it was never enough to generate an effective immune response strong enough to eliminate the cancer. That is because cancer grows from the healthy cells in our body, so it can easily trick the immune system into thinking the cancer belongs there. Even more troubling, once it does so, it can turn the immune system against itself, causing immune cells to kill other immune cells that want to attack the cancer. This is a key concept to understand: The immune system has cells that are called "regulatory cells," which are designed to protect you from autoimmunity, a condition caused by your immune system attacking yourself. But these regulatory cells can be high jacked by cancer and used as its personal bodyguards. When this happens, it is these regulatory cells that often are the most important barrier to an anti-cancer immune response. Blocking or destroying these regulatory immune cells is one of the key features to the more successful immunotherapy drugs.

In essence, as powerful as the immune system is, cancer has been even more intelligent. It is not just the fact that the immune system fails to recognize cancer that has made cancer so challenging to treat effectively, but also the fact that cancer is actively able to avoid the immune system.

In simple terms, you can think of the immune system as having two main divisions, one designed to attack harmful foreign substances and the other to protect against an overzealous immune response, acting as defense against "autoimmunity"—the process of immune cells misperceiving cells in the body as foreign invaders and attacking them by mistake. I stress this again because it is important: The division designed to protect the body from a mistaken immune attack is known as the regulatory immune system. The regulatory immune system is obviously critical to reduce the risk of autoimmune diseases which arise when the immune system thinks the body's own cells are foreign ones and must be destroyed. The regulatory immune system helps prevent these mistaken attacks on the body's own cells. You can think of the protective, regulatory side of the immune system as being the "brakes" and the attacking side as being the "gas pedal." No matter how much you push the gas, if the brakes are fully applied you will go nowhere. Unfortunately, what that means when it comes to cancer is that the regulatory portion of the immune system prevents the rest of the immune system from attacking cancer cells because those cells are masquerading as normal, natural cells that belong there. Thus, failing to recognize the cancer cells for what they are, the regulatory immune system is an important protector of cancer.

Despite these challenges, the concept of teaching the immune system to recognize cancer and destroy it has seemed like the best chance to create a cure in a high percentage of cancer patients. The immune system has its own intelligence and it has memory, both of which are crucial to seek out and kill cancer. A good immune response recognizes many targets on a cancer, so-called cancer antigens, making it harder for the cancer to hide. This is the weakness with some of the one-dimensional treatments, which includes some vaccines and original versions of CAR-T, which generally target one antigen. Later in this book, I will discuss in more detail how intra-tumoral immunotherapy, the injection of immunotherapy directly into a cancer, may be a good solution to this problem.

Given this complexity of the immune response, indiscriminately enhancing the immune system in an effort to treat cancer may not always be a good idea because doing so could strengthen the regulatory system's protections against autoimmunity, and thus protect the cancer cells.

On the other hand, it is well known that chemotherapy weakens the immune system, which is often considered a bad side effect. But certain chemotherapy drugs may also weaken the regulatory immune system, which may in turn enhance the anti-cancer response of the immune system. For this reason, medications are often used to reduce the regulatory cells of the immune system, which seem more susceptible to certain chemotherapy agents. Low dose cyclophosphamide is one of these. However it is important to point out that it is "low dose" and usually does not have the typical side effects as when used as a high dose "chemotherapy" agent. Most patients should not have any of the side effects that they would experience with standard chemotherapy type doses.

Are you sufficiently confused? You should be. Cancer and cancer treatment is confusing given the complexity of the immune system. But what all this means in a nutshell is that the immune system attacks foreign bodies—we call this the "effector response"—while the regulatory portion of the immune system prevents it from attacking itself. Because cancer disguises itself as a natural part of the body, the regulatory system gets fooled and protects the cancer. It lets cancer cells grow, thinking they belong there. Compounding this problem, these regulatory cells may often produce substances to assist the cancer in growing and suppressing the "effector" anti-cancer immune attack. Typically cancer cannot survive, or at least thrive, without the help of the regulatory immune cells. These regulatory immune cells become accomplices to the cancer. As they say, "With friends like that, who needs enemies."

The challenge to successful immunotherapy has been to override the regulatory system, while at the same time strengthening the rest of the immune system. And that challenge has been nearly insurmountable. Until recently.

In the mid-1990's, Dr. James Allison, Chairman of Immunology at the University of Texas, MD Anderson Cancer Center, discovered some of the key mechanisms that result in putting on the "brakes" of the immune system. Dr. Allison had long been a pioneer in the study of T cells, cells that are fundamental to the immune response. Think of T cells as the immune system's soldiers, the "killer T cells" which attack foreign invaders. There is another type of T cell called a "helper T cell" which organizes and helps other cells do their job in the immune system.

These T cells, along with other immune cells, contain receptors that can activate regulatory T cells (called Tregs), which determine if something is friend or foe. If these regulatory T cells determine something is foreign and dangerous, signals are released to stimulate an attacking immune response. If, on the other hand, they identify it as a "friend," the regulatory T cells tell the immune system to back off.

But as I've said, cancer cells have corresponding receptors which send deceptive signals to the regulatory T cells to trick them into thinking they are "friends" and a natural part of the body not to be attacked. Dr. Allison's understanding of this process led to the development of a series of drugs known as immune checkpoint inhibitors. Essentially, these drugs inhibit the immune checkpoint response by removing cancer's disguise. By blocking this signal, the immune system can potentially see the cancer for what it really is, something dangerous and that needs to be destroyed because it doesn't belong in your body.

Based on Dr. Allison's research, in March 2011, the FDA approved a drug called Ipilimumab, more commonly known by its brand name, Yervoy, for the treatment of melanoma. The approval of this exciting new drug, which helps remove the brakes of the regulatory immune system, unleashing the attacking side to go after the cancer, heralded a change in thinking that began a revolution in cancer treatment. A key weakness had been discovered, and even though the initial immune checkpoint inhibitors may not be the ultimate cure in their own right, they have certainly lit the way.

More significantly, after the development of this first immune checkpoint inhibitor drug, researchers realized that removing the "brakes" of the immune system was a key step in coaxing the immune system to unleash the body's own defense system against the cancer. This has led to a new understanding in cancer treatment, and many future drug therapies. The potential for immunotherapy to become a leading treatment for a variety of cancers is now within our sights, and for many patients they have already proven lifesaving.

I would be remiss if I didn't also mention Tasuku Honjo, MD, PhD, and his work researching a protein known as programmed cell death protein 1 (PD-1). PD-1 is found on the surface of cells. Like regulatory T cells, its function is to regulate the immune system's response to other human cells, thus also preventing autoimmunity by minimizing T cell inflammatory activity.

However, also like regulatory T cells, PD-1 can prevent the immune system from recognizing and killing cancer cells. Dr. Honjo's study of PD-1 led to the development of a new class of drugs called PD-1 inhibitors. At present, they are the most widely used immunotherapy drugs. Both Drs. Allison and Honjo were awarded the 2018 Nobel Prize in Physiology or Medicine for their work that led to the development of immune checkpoint inhibitors.

Since approval of Yervoy, several other important new drugs have been approved by the FDA. The current, most popular immune checkpoint inhibitors in clinical use are Ipilimumab (trade name Yervoy), Nivolumab and Pembrozolumab (under the trade names Opdivo and Keytruda, respectively). On May 18, 2016, the FDA approved Atezolizumab (under the brand name Tecentriq) for treatment of bladder cancer. Since then other PD-1/PD-L1 drugs have been approved, as well. There are many other drugs that are in development and will probably soon gain approval, but for now, these drugs are our primary medications used in immunotherapy, and will be an important focus of this book.

Before going any further, there are a few key concepts that you need to understand if you or someone you love is considering immunotherapy.

1. It does not always matter what type of cancer you have, there can be a potential for immunotherapy to work.

Early efforts to treat cancer had assumed that cancer was cancer. But we now know that there are over two hundred different types of cancer. That means what works for one form of cancer may not work for others. But don't let that fact discourage you. One of the most exciting features of immunotherapy is that, because it works in conjunction with the body's natural immune system, it has the potential to treat many types of cancer, and hopefully, as new drugs are developed, maybe all cancers. Different cancers may have their specific immune weaknesses, and those are being rapidly sorted out with current immunotherapy research.

Unfortunately, I often hear from patients who have been told by their doctor that immunotherapy does not work for their cancer type. I think if you look at the research, however, and the swift pace at which immunotherapy is gaining approval, you will agree that it is probably not true. I do admit that the current CTLA-4/PD-1/PD-L1 drugs may still be lacking. While it is true that some cancers are more immunogenic and respond better than others to immunotherapy, there is the potential for *all* cancers to respond to immunotherapy—particularly when used in combinations, directly injected into the tumor, or together with ablation procedures in a specific manner. I have many patients with lung cancer, bladder cancer and kidney cancer who were told that immunotherapy drugs would not work for their cancer, but now these same drugs have been approved for those cancer types. Because it takes years of research before the FDA will approve a specific drug for a specific form of cancer, the FDA approval process is a slow one.

While drugs cannot be prescribed in the U.S. without having been approved by the FDA, once approved for use for one condition, FDA approval is not necessary for a physician to prescribe that drug for a condition for which it has not been approved. This is known as off-label use and is quite common. That means that while Yervoy was first approved for the treatment of melanoma, physicians can still prescribe it to treat other cancers.

2. Typically your health insurance will not cover the costs of the drugs without FDA approval for your specific form of cancer, but combining immunotherapy with cryoablation or directly injecting the drugs into the tumor can drastically reduce the costs of medications.

Unfortunately, insurance carriers will almost never provide coverage for a drug used to treat a condition that the FDA hasn't approved it to treat. That means that if the drug your physician prescribes has not been approved by the FDA to treat the specific form of cancer you have, it may be almost impossible for him or her to offer you a standard immunotherapy treatment that is not directly covered by insurance, even if it may work. Yervoy, for example, may be covered by your insurance carrier for treating certain cases of melanoma, but not for treating other cancers. With a price tag at over $30,000 per infusion—and a course of treatment requiring a minimum of four infusions—it remains a treatment that many patients cannot afford. Bristol-Myers Squibb, the makers of Yervoy, does offer a patient-assistance program that may reduce cost, but it may still be such a steep price beyond the reach of many. There is also the difficulty of finding doctors who may be willing to offer these medications "off-label." Also keep in mind that we are mainly discussing advanced, Stage IV patients, for which standard therapies may have failed or been of limited success.

Even though the drugs are available outside the United States, where in most cases they would be much less expensive than they are in the U.S., immunotherapy pricing remains fairly steep throughout the world.

But don't let the price of these drugs discourage you. The key aspect to injecting the drugs directly into the tumor, rather than into the bloodstream, means that even without ablation, it may be possible to achieve the same or better results with a fraction of the dose—and at a fraction of the costs.[34] In other words, whereas standard immunotherapy treatment involves infusing the drugs into the bloodstream, by combining immunotherapy with cryoablation or directly injecting these medications into the tumor, the effectiveness of the treatment may be enhanced while the price of that treatment is dramatically reduced.

3. Combination immunotherapy is generally more effective than any single agent.

The anti-cancer immune response is as complex as is cancer itself. It is highly unlikely that one agent alone is sufficient to generate an effective anti-cancer immune response. Not only does CTLA-4 help tumors to suppress the immune response against them, PD-1 also plays an important role.

It has already been shown in clinical trials that the combination of anti-CTLA-4 and anti-PD-1 inhibitors is significantly more effective than either one alone. Just recently the FDA has added approvals of this combination for certain melanoma, kidney and colon cancers. Unfortunately, just as success increases, so does the cost and side effects of the two drugs just as significantly. This is one reason that we inject the medications into the tumor microenvironment, where they need to be. You want the immune response to be directed against the tumor, and where that is more likely to occur is at the tumor site. Once the immune system "learns" how to respond in one location, it is better able to attack cancer elsewhere in the body.

In addition, a treatment such as cryoablation, which is the direct freezing of the tumor, has its own immune-stimulating properties. It can be considered an additional form of immunotherapy to be used with immune checkpoint inhibitors. And because ablation is minimally invasive and tumors are treated with a needle under image guidance, it is the perfect opportunity to administer other immune agents, such as the checkpoint inhibitor drugs, directly into the tumor, at the same time, in one procedure.

Throughout the history of modern medicine, we have found many remarkable powerhouse treatment combinations. A great example is the treatment of HIV/AIDS. Just a few decades ago, an HIV diagnosis was a terminal one. But the current medications used today in combination have had great success and patients can live long, relatively normal lives with their disease. But when these same drugs are used alone, there is only a modest survival increase. Hence, the lessons we have learned in treating HIV patients supports the importance of combination therapy in treating disease, and cancer is no different.

Immune checkpoint inhibitors not only help unlock a natural immune response, they can be essential for helping other immune therapies turn from bust to boom. It's that synergistic immune response that enables cancer treatments to become far more effective than ever before. While our knowledge of immunotherapy is still developing, we have finally reached a point where cancer patients—like former President Jimmy Carter—can recover from malignant and fast-growing tumors previously thought hopeless. And when I talk about hope, I'm not talking about just passively sitting back and hoping for a cure. I'm talking about taking charge of the recovery process by doing everything possible to give the immune system a fighting chance against cancer.

CHAPTER 3

Cancer and the Immune System

T HERE IS A very complex interplay between cancer and the immune system. This involves many cell types. We still have much to understand, but it is useful to know the basic mechanisms, so that potential treatments can be understood.

When you think of cancer, it is best to consider it like a well-organized terrorist group. In this analogy, your body is a country, like the U.S. You are the President. Cancer has invaded your country and infiltrated into your people. You cannot always tell who they are by looking at them. The terrorist (cancer) has many ways it can attack you. In addition, it is spreading its message, trying to convert some of your citizens (normal cells) to work for it. These are your normal native-born citizens, but the cancer can convince them that its ideas are correct, and you and your government are wrong. Obviously there is a minority of these people that can be converted to the enemy, but when converted they can use the fact that they are insiders to their advantage. This story has many characters you might see in a war on terrorism. Here is the overview of characters:

Your country (your body).

President:	You. You are the leader of your body and make the decisions of potential actions against the terrorist in hopes to keep your citizens safe and ensure the survival of your country.
Minister of Defense:	Your healthcare team/doctor. They advise you, but it is up to you as the president to make the final decisions.
Terrorist group:	Cancer. It is well organized and as it grows it has more power and funding.
Immune system:	The military/police/homeland security. It is made up of many groups of agents with different functions.

Once the cancer terrorist group has invaded your country, when it is small or isolated, it is easier to control and prevent major damage. However, once it grows in power, it is much more difficult to control. The problem is that your own agents can be converted over to help the cancer. Not just your normal citizens, but your military as well. This is always something that I think is very surprising to patients: Your own cells and immune system can and will betray you. Two of the most notorious that you need to know about are called myeloid-derived suppressor cells (MDSCs) and tumor-associated macrophages (TAMs). There are two types of TAMs: M1 and M2. M1 TAMs attack cancer, while M2 protects and helps it. To effectively fight cancer you need to decrease the MDSCs and M2 type TAMs.

In addition, some of your normal citizen cells can act like sympathizers, assisting the cancer to grow. These are often some of your tissue support cells, called stroma. Stroma may help hide the cancer and provide it food and other substances that cancer needs to survive.

As you learned in Chapter 2, included in your immune system are T effector cells and T regulatory cells (Tregs). Continuing our analogy, T effector cells act like attack drones. However, they need permission to unleash their attack. The T regulatory cells (Tregs) are the ones that give this permission. However, the Tregs do not have the killer instinct like your T effector attackers. In order to protect against casualties of normal citizens (an autoimmune response), they keep a leash on your T attackers. The Tregs also are being tricked by the terrorists (cancer cells), so they are hesitant to unleash an attack on them. However, if you can decrease the number of Treg cells, the T attackers can be unleashed to go after the terrorists. However, it is not always so easy. You need to know where your terrorists are located. You need intelligence on them. You cannot attack something that you cannot identify. There are the old ways of poisoning them with chemo or nuking them with radiation, but that generally just causes them to change location and results in a lot of collateral damage. You need a more precise attack, like a strike drone that can take them out with little normal casualties. For this, you need to give your T attackers good intel. They need to know where the terrorists are and what they look like. Then you need to get your personnel in the right location. It does no good if your soldiers want to attack, but they are not in the right spot. Your immune system may want to attack cancer, but it needs to know where to go.

Your immune system also includes immune cells known as antigen presenting cells, one example of which is the dendritic cell. It acts like a spy gathering intel and providing it to your immune system. But if the dendritic cells have bad information, they can lead your T attackers astray. Without the correct information, dendritic cells are more likely to slow your immune system down than to help it. For this reason, the use of dendritic therapy alone to treat cancer has been disappointing.

These are the basics of mounting a good assault and eliminating the terrorists.

The President needs to make good decision based on intel from the advisors. Ultimately it is the President that will be held accountable should the war be lost.

The Minister of Defense needs to provide the President with the best information possible from the team of experts.

Cells that are going to hinder the ability of your attackers need to be decreased. This means decreasing MDSCs, Tregs and TAMs. However, in regards to TAMs, it is even better if you can convert them to your side (M1 type).

Your attackers need to know where the cancer is located and want to attack it. Often, the cancer is so sneaky, it has infiltrated and is living in your body undetected by the immune system's "surveillance system". Even if you use some of your new immunotherapy weapons, those are not effective enough. First, you must alert your attackers where the cancer is located, then, you signal for it to attack with FDA-approved immunotherapy drugs. Unfortunately, most of the time your attackers do not have enough intel, so traditional immunotherapy, as good as it may be, fails far more than it succeeds. So, it is up to you to provide it with the tools of success. In addition, newer weapons and technology are going to provide your attackers with the means necessary to hunt down the enemy and destroy them.

One such weapon is cryoablation. The use of this therapy is like destroying a small terrorist cell while also gathering the motherlode of intel. Then you can use that intel to flush out and destroy your enemy (cancer) throughout your country (body).

Just as a one-dimensional attack is very unlikely to rid your country of terrorists, so too is the one-dimensional approach of "cut, poison, and burn" that is traditional cancer therapy unlikely to achieve lasting remission. True success often requires the interplay of many anti-cancer agents working together to address the complex multiple factors that cause cancer. This one-dimensional attack remains the weakness in most traditional cancer treatment approaches, including traditional immunotherapy. It is up to you, as the President, to make sure that your country is provided with all of the weapons necessary to win this war. In the rest of this book you will learn more about each of these weapons and why, together, they offer the best solution for defeating cancer.

CHAPTER 4

AblationVax™:
The Cancer Ablation
"Vaccine"

I CANNOT IMAGINE EVEN one cancer patient who would not be excited about the idea of having their cancer successfully treated by just inserting a needle into a malignant tumor and destroying it directly. As previously discussed, image-guided cancer ablation involves using computed tomography (CT) or ultrasound to help the physician guide a needle through the body and insert it directly into the tumor. The tumor can then be directly destroyed by either heating it with microwaves or radiofrequency, or by freezing it through cryoablation. The idea sounds so simple, yet few patients know that this treatment is an option. We are now able to directly freeze or burn many tumors without removing them.

Why wouldn't we just remove them? Well it turns out that one of the keys to successful immunotherapy is leaving the destroyed tumor in the body. This is how our immune system can gather intel about the cancer to more effectively fight it.

Though I am mainly going to discuss how the powerful combination of cryoablation and immunotherapy works well for treating advanced cancers, it is also increasingly being considered for treating early stage cancer, as well, especially in cases of breast, lung, and liver cancer, where ablation is being looked at as a future surgery replacement. I expect to see cryoablation used more frequently in early stage cancer, along with immune-enhancing measures to reduce the risk of future metastasis.

When cancer moves beyond its very early stages, it is systemic—and can spread throughout the body. After primary tumors are removed by surgery, cancer patients are often told, "We got all of it." This isn't true. Even if you remove the primary tumor, cancer cells still remain and are able to proliferate and form new tumors over time. In cases of advanced cancer, when a tumor is killed by ablation, the dead cancer cells act like a vaccine, causing the immune response to kick in to attack foreign bodies, including remaining cancer cells in the body. However, this does not usually happen without a little help from some type of immunotherapy.

Hardly anyone, including doctors who perform this procedure, realize that cryoablation can be used to generate a powerful immune response leading to one of the most successful cancer treatments that exist, particularly for patients with Stage III or IV cancer, where the options for treatment are most limited. Each year there are approximately 600,000 advanced cancers diagnosed in the U.S., which would otherwise be practically hopeless cases. But with this ablation technique, combined with immunotherapy, we now have the chance to save many of those lives. Moreover, patients with earlier stages of cancer who would otherwise suffer through toxic chemotherapy and radiation now have more effective choices of treatment with far fewer side effects. I like to call this combination therapy AblationVax™ because of how it optimizes the body's immune system, similar to how vaccines do.

When I was in medical school and early residency and learned about the potential of this technique to treat cancer, I thought it was the most amazing thing I had heard and assumed word of this new strategy would spread quickly and all oncologists would jump on board. I recognized that the future of cancer treatment would be to target the tumor directly using minimally invasive techniques and image guidance, but I have since discovered that these ablation techniques have been slow to catch on. Even now, years later, the techniques are vastly under-utilized.

The reluctance of oncologists to treat patients with cryoablation and immunotherapy (AblationVax™) may be because health insurance does not always cover it, and few physicians want to engage in treatment plans that are costly, not covered by insurance, and remain relatively new. Moreover, oncologists who oversee and control most of the cancer care their patients receive are not trained in cryoablation and lack the necessary skill to perform the procedure. And I cannot imagine that any oncologist would be excited about giving up control of cancer treatment to the radiologist, as it would surely lead to the end of their specialty.

It is for these reasons, I believe, that this procedure may not take off until the oncologists themselves learn to do it. This is much like treating atherosclerotic heart disease with coronary angioplasty. This procedure was invented by the radiologist Charles Dotter in 1964. While coronary angioplasty is extremely common today, it did not take off until the mid to late 1980's. Prior to that time, radiologists had been performing the procedures and cardiologists were reluctant to recommend them. Once cardiologists started doing them, however, they became routine. Also, I might add, insurance coverage for the procedure helped, as well. Over time, I am confident that this reluctance by oncologists to use cryoablation will change.

Image-guided ablation when done correctly can stimulate an anti-cancer immune response, although when done alone it is generally not curative outside of cases of limited disease or early cancer. However, I would like to add food for thought here. What if the earlier stage patients that we treat with ablation also had some immune-stimulating agents added as well? How many cancers would we prevent from ever becoming advanced in the first place? I would say that most could be, and it is of course the advanced cancers that are the real killers.

I suspect that most, if not all, doctors performing ablation procedures do not fully understand how it interacts with the immune response. The type of ablation technique used (whether freezing through cryoablation or heating through microwaves and radiofrequency), and the tumor size are some of the key aspects to creating an effective immune response. The combination of immunotherapy and ablation is highly effective, but each of these therapies must be done simultaneously for them to be effective. Studies by Den Brok show that the timing of immunotherapy procedures is also critical. In other words, not all ablation is created equal and when not administered correctly it can be harmful if it leads to enhancement of the regulatory immune system—thinking the tumor belongs there—and allows the cancer cells to flourish. Because so few doctors are trained and experienced in achieving the best combination of these treatments, most are unfamiliar with—if not hostile to—ablation and immunotherapy treatments.

And unfortunately, since cancer patients are customers who provide their livelihood, far too many oncologists are hesitant to admit they lack the skill to treat their patients with these advanced techniques, and thus they are reluctant to refer them to someone else who may be able to do better, particularly if they haven't had any direct experience with what they might regard as an experimental technique. The radiologist relies mostly on referrals from other doctors, so they certainly do not want to upset their oncologist, who can be a major referrer. Even though there are many skilled radiologists who could do this procedure, there is not enough to service the potential future demand of this and other image-guided cancer procedures when these techniques take off. Though our scientific understanding of ablation continues to advance, I think it will take oncologists learning to do this procedure for the therapy to become more widely available. Unfortunately, this requires many years of training in imaging and image-guided procedures, which is a real barrier to entry. However, just as cardiologists have done a great job getting into image-guided heart procedures, I am sure that oncologists can do it as well. It may just add some years to their training, just like it did in cardiology. I certainly welcome this and will be glad to train them when the time comes. It is time for a paradigm shift in the treatment of cancer, and our loyalty must be to curing the patient, not to the future of any particular medical specialty. It is only a matter of time that these jobs will be done by robots and A.I. (artificial intelligence) anyway.

At this time, in our profit-oriented medical system, there is little incentive for oncologists to encourage cryoablation immunotherapy (AblationVax™) for their patients, and most cancer patients remain uninformed of the breakthroughs we have had, particularly for those with advanced stage cancer.

In our early efforts to treat patients through cryoablation and immunotherapy, it was initially thought that the patients who would have the most success were those whose cancer was discovered at an early stage—before it had spread through the body. When I first began doing ablation procedures, some 16+ years ago, I felt that even among those with advanced disease, if I could reduce tumor bulk by fifty to seventy percent, that it would be a huge success. Even if I did not cure those patients, I could give them precious added months or even years to live—without the wretched side effects of radiation and chemotherapy. Yet when I discussed my views with many of my colleagues, I was startled to find that few shared my views. The consensus was that we should focus on the patients with the best chance at survival—those with Stage I and Stage II cancers. A fifty to seventy percent reduction in tumor bulk was not considered much of a success for advanced patients. Yet, had any chemotherapy been capable of the same reduction in tumor bulk, it would be considered very successful. There seemed to be two dueling standards of success among my colleagues—one for the tried and true chemotherapy, and the other for the new and growing field of research in radiofrequency and cryoablation. We were the new kids on the block, and the old guard was wary.

Undaunted, I began taking on many cases that others considered too advanced or hopeless to bother with. These were the patients who often had no other options. My philosophy was, if it was myself, and there was something that at least had a chance of helping me, I would take it. I also felt that it was just common sense—less cancer is better, at least if it didn't bring more misery. Certainly when fighting a war, when you reduce the number of your enemy, you are making progress.

I was optimistic, but unprepared for how successful my approach proved to be. While many patients did die from their advanced disease, a fair number of the patients who came to me with Stage III and Stage IV cancers did far better than I ever could have imagined. One key thing that I observed was that rarely, but significantly, a patient's non-treated tumors would shrink or disappear after another tumor had been treated. This was what had happened with my colleague's mother, who I discussed in Chapter One. We had only treated the tumors in one lung, yet the tumors in the other lung had disappeared by the time of her next visit.

A similar and much more remarkable case encouraged me even further. In 2003, a gentleman from Atlanta, Georgia contacted me, hoping I would consider performing ablation. He had metastatic melanoma, with more than thirty lesions in one of his lungs, and his death was imminent. I had to tell him that he had too many lesions and I did not feel ablation would help. Asking me to reconsider, he said he just had a strong belief that ablation was the answer. Still, I declined, again explaining that his cancer was far too advanced. But he was persistent, rejecting my logic and appealing to my emotions. He told me that his doctors had told him that he had only one to three months to live, but his daughter was getting married in five months and he wanted to walk her down the aisle. He was certain that ablation would give him the extra time he needed to see his daughter get married. How could I possibly deny this man the one chance he thought would help, even if I felt otherwise?

I agreed to perform the ablation, but I was frank with him and told him I still didn't think it would help. I told him my plan was to ablate as much as possible in a series of procedures because his tumors were so numerous that it would not be possible to ablate them all in a single procedure. There was not a realistic way to ablate all the tumors, but I think I even convinced myself that my motto of "less cancer is always better" would hold true in his case as well.

Satisfied that I would at least give him the chance he sought, he agreed to my plan. Shortly after, I performed the first ablation without any problems, as is typical for ablation, and asked him to return in a month for a second procedure, not certain he would make it that long.

But a month later, he did return and we performed a CT scan to assess the progression of the tumors to prepare for the next procedure. As the images came across the computer, I could not believe my eyes. The lesions were gone, all of them. We had not touched the other lesions, yet they had disappeared.

I wept, realizing in that moment that I had just witnessed something amazing, something that would change the history of cancer treatment, perhaps even turn out to be the greatest advance in cancer treatment to date. It was something so simple. We did not have to cut people open to remove their tumors. Just like a biopsy, we could simply insert a needle into a tumor and heat or freeze it to destroy it directly.

The discovery was almost too good to be true. It had been a childhood dream of mine, since my grandmother's illness and death, to cure cancer. I had so wanted to make my grandmother proud, to somehow avenge her death by catching her killer—and to save countless other lives. And here it was, staring me in the face in the form of these CT scan images. What had been over thirty lesions had miraculously disappeared. It was better than winning the lottery a thousand times over. I thought, out of all the possible areas I could have been involved in medicine, in cancer, could I have been lucky enough to pick the right one, a legitimate road to a cure?

About a year after treating this gentleman from Atlanta, he contacted me again. His cancer had unfortunately returned, though it was not quite as bad as before. He asked me if I could try the same procedure once more. It had enabled him to achieve his goal of walking his daughter down the aisle. But now there was another goal. His daughter was pregnant, and she was due in several months. Could I help him to see the birth of his first grandchild?

Of course, this time, I didn't have to put much thought into it. We performed the procedure and once again, within a month, the visible lesions in his lung were gone. But the success was bittersweet. Having succeeded in eliminating them the first time, only to have them return shortly after, I knew that the challenge before me was not just to eliminate the tumors, but to make sure they didn't return. And how could I ensure that the success we had with one gentleman could be repeated with others? How could I ensure that the response was the same for other advanced cases?

As time went on, the answers to these questions would become more evident, but it would take nearly another decade of research and practice. In the meantime, my patient did live to see the birth of his grandchild, and I hope, to see other birthdays, as well. Unfortunately, I was unable to keep treating him due to hospital and insurance policies, limiting our use of ablation outside very limited areas. I moved on to another hospital and the patient and I lost touch after a couple more years. While I am almost certain that his cancer did return, I feel better just thinking that there is a chance that he is still alive after all these years. I am, however, confident that if we had the weapons then that we have now, he would still be alive to see his grandchildren graduate and marry.

Even if his cancer did return, one thing I am certain of is that his treatment was not in vain. Not only was he able to have at least three more years of good health after being given a prognosis of one to three months, the amazing success of his ablation procedure kept me going whenever I became discouraged, and it keeps me going today. Ablation had triggered a powerful immune response that eliminated over two dozen tumors without even touching them.

Those rare but fascinating responses were what led me to suspect an immune response, similar to a vaccine, had been set in action by the ablation process. Ablation kills tumors in the body and leaves dead pieces, known as antigens, for the immune system to recognize. This is providing the intel your immune cells need to know what to look for to find the enemy. Also, what is now known is that ablation creates an inflammatory process that is also immune-stimulating, what we call "Danger Signals." These are some of the signals to attract your immune cells (attackers) to the location of the bad guys.

In fact, when you look at the immune aspects, ablation can be a very effective stimulus of the the body's overall anti-cancer immune response.

Another huge advantage to ablation is just reducing tumor bulk, so that immunotherapy and the anti-cancer immune response have a weaker opponent to attack. By reducing the size of the tumor, the patient has a better theoretical chance of immunotherapy working. In our war on terrorism model, ablation reduces the number of your enemy, weakening them, giving you access to intel which helps to better recognize, locate, and eliminate the terrorist.

Though these early successes were significant and exciting findings, triggering the immune response to attack untreated tumors remained elusive. I was finding great success with the cryoablation technique on the tumors that I destroyed directly, but I wanted to determine how we could make this happen in almost every case. The initial answer, as it turned out, was in immune checkpoint inhibitors. Though these drugs combined with ablation may not be perfect, they were a huge advancement.

Remember that the immune checkpoints are the key "braking" mechanism of the immune system. And no matter how much you step on the gas, when the brakes are applied you will go nowhere. Well we have recently discovered, through some key animal research, that there is massive synergy between immune checkpoint inhibitors and ablation. We still need continued research in this area, but most studies point to cryoablation being more immune-stimulating than other ablative techniques such as radiofrequency and microwave ablation, which are heat-based. The main theory is that cryoablation, as it kills tumors, leaves more tumor pieces, "antigens", attack to be recognized by the immune system. This is certainly true, though there are several other aspects as well, but I will not burden you with the scientific details. In our war on terrorism analogy, you want to destroy the tumor, but leave evidence and other supplies intact, to use as intel to locate the other terrorists. If you blow everything to pieces, you destroy valuable information for tracking them down. If you kill with freezing, there will be more intact pieces than if you burn the place down.

Continuing my quest to find a better solution, I began combining image-guided ablation, usually cryoablation, with the approved immune checkpoint inhibitors that were available at that time, Keytruda and Yervoy.

One of the first cases we did with ablation and Keytruda was with a patient we will call LS. Her cancer was very advanced, with diffuse lesions of the lung and bones, and of the brain, as well. Though what we did is very limited compared to what we do now, the amazing thing in her case is that not only did we see the lesions throughout her body disappear, but most (unfortunately not all) of her brain lesions went away. Shortly after Keytruda and Yervoy were approved, another PD-1 inhibitor, Opdivo, was approved for cancer treatment. We found that our success was enhanced by treating patients with a single drug in combination with the ablation, but when we gave them a combination of two or more of the drugs along with the ablation the results were astounding. I think the combination of ablation and immunotherapy had been the biggest advance in cancer treatment in human history at that time, although today it has probably been supplanted by the combination of OX40/CpG/Yervoy. I am hopeful that with this drug combination, along with new drugs that are continuing to be developed and approved, we will soon see a treatment that will cure the majority of cancer patients. One important aspect with ablation is that there are certain techniques which can make the difference between a positive anti-cancer immune response and no response. In some cases, the wrong technique can even hinder the anti-cancer immune response. Cryoablation tends to be more immune-stimulating than other techniques, but if the physician ablates too much at one time the immune response may actually be inhibited, causing other tumors to grow faster. It is important for any physician performing cryoablation to understand how much is too much in order to create the best immune response. Some studies suggest that not ablating the entire tumor may be immunologically superior to ablating the entire tumor. There is probably a lot of variability on what is the exact size and volume of tumor to ablate. We have a better understanding now that there are indications that overzealous ablation, or ablation of too much normal tissue, which occurs when trying to obtain clean margins, may actually be harmful in the long run. It seems that these aspects may lead to an increased healing response, with release of growth factors and immune suppressive substances, like TGF-B, HGF and VEGF. The techniques that we work with to enhance the immune response are related to reducing or actively blocking these substances. It has also been identified that these same aspects occur in standard surgery as well, and may lead to the increase in future cancer spread. In surgery, the use of Ketorolac, an anti-inflammatory drug, has been shown to reduce some of this risk. We use Ketorolac injected into the ablation site, hopefully reducing this risk. I would like to add here that not only should Ketorolac be considered with surgery or ablation to reduce future spread of cancer, but for biopsies as well because the growth factors stimulated by surgery and ablation can also occur from biopsies. I find that it is important not to ablate too much tumor and certainly little to no normal tissue if possible. This only applies to advanced disease. When I am treating someone with only local early stage disease it is necessary to ablate the entire tumor, with a margin, to reduce the risk of local recurrence. This is the same concept as surgical removal. However, when dealing with advanced disease, we are going to need an immune response if we hope to obtain a cure, so we perform the cryoablation using techniques to enhance the immune response. Though we are still learning what this may entail, our current understanding is that ablating too much tumor volume, too much normal tissue, or ablating at a slow rate of freeze-all probably hurt the potential immune response.

Often patients ask if surgery or ablation alone could be used for advanced disease. Though there may be certain exceptions, generally you would not do these procedures alone because in its advanced stage cancer is systemic and requires a systemic treatment. For advanced cancer, I do not use ablation alone. It is always combined with immunotherapy injected into the ablated tumor. This is a systemic treatment.

I have found that heat-based ablations (using microwaves or radiofrequency) are immune-stimulating, but probably not to the level that can be generated by freezing the tumor through cryoablation. But heat-based ablations seem to have less negative impact on the immune response for treating larger tumors, so they remain good techniques for reducing the size of large tumors. When we are dealing with large tumor bulk, reduction in size can be obtained with a heat-based ablation, then we can perform cryoablation on a smaller area of tumor in order to enhance the immune response. This is done in conjunction with the injection of immunotherapy into the cryoablation tumor site. This combination of techniques effectively delivers a one-two punch to the tumor and provides a powerful immune-stimulating response. We are already working on drug techniques to eliminate any negative immune effects and further accentuate the positive aspects. It is possible new drugs may even eliminate the need for ablation all together. Further research in this area will certainly lead to new changes in techniques and likely the devices we use to do the procedures as well.

Research conducted by Dr. Michael S. Sabel at the University of Michigan has shown that the rate of freeze is very important for the immune response. Basically Dr. Sabel showed that faster freezing was immune-stimulating, while slower freezing was immune suppressing. For this reason, we changed the cryoablation device that we use, which previously was an argon gas-based system, to a liquid nitrogen-based system (IceSense3, IceCure) which has a faster rate of freeze. This system was originally designed for the breast, but now can treat anywhere in the body that cryoablation can typically be performed. Most cryoablation done in the U.S. (and probably most of the world) is performed with argon-based systems, which may freeze at a slower rate. These systems are subject to changes in freeze rate based on the available gas pressures. One important aspect that I have observed with argon-based systems is that as you are doing the procedure, the pressure of argon in your tank will decrease. Ultimately as the procedure goes on, you will have to change tanks to maintain pressure. As the pressure decreases, so does the rate of freeze. For me, this further adds reason to using a liquid nitrogen-based system, where the rate of freeze remains constant. Certainly more research needs to be done in this area, but I think the work by Dr. Sabel is extremely helpful. This is enough information for me at the moment to only use a system that is known to freeze at a faster rate that remains constant throughout the procedure.

In addition to injecting immune checkpoint inhibitor drugs in and around the ablated tumors, there are also numerous vaccine adjuvants that can be used. Adjuvants are substances which help stimulate the immune response further. Standard vaccinations, such as the flu, often include an adjuvant because the killed virus or virus pieces alone are often not sufficient enough to generate immunity. The same goes with cancer. There are many different adjuvant agents available to enhance the immune response. As I mentioned before, the excellent research by Den Brok, et al. from the Netherlands has shown significantly improved results with reduced future metastasis and recurrence (in the animal model) when combining cryoablation of a tumor with direct injection of Saponin, which is a soap-like substance that comes from the soap bark tree in Chile. There is a commercially available modified form of this made by Novavax called Matrix M. Basically these adjuvants enhance the delivery of the tumor pieces (antigens) to the immune system and dendritic cells. We have also used Montanide ISA 51 made by Seppic, this is an oil/water vaccine adjuvant, which, in addition to being an adjuvant, it also seems to cause a slow release delivery of the directly injected immunotherapy agents, such as the immune checkpoint inhibitors. One key aspect is that it is very helpful to mix the immunotherapy agents with something that helps keep it in the local tumor environment. We often use either Montanide ISA 51 or a hydrogel to achieve a depot effect in the tumor microenvironment. If you inject just a water-soluble drug, especially in a non-ablated tumor, much of the drug may exit the tumor microenvironment due to the increased blood flow often found with tumors, creating a wash out effect. This is less of an issue injecting into an ablated tumor, as usually the blood flow has been cut off or reduced by the ablation process. This is another advantage offered by ablation. However, I still feel it is good to use an agent that will cause a slow release and keep the medication for an extended period of time within the tumor environment.

Without going into too much detail of the science behind these findings (which you can find in the References), the basic process involves killing the tumor with cryoablation that will simultaneously stimulate the immune system, and adding vaccine adjuvants and immune checkpoint inhibitor drugs directly at the ablation site so that the typical aspects that will inhibit an effective immune response are blocked. This process creates an effective tumor "vaccine" which, while not technically a vaccine against cancer that healthy people can use to protect against cancer cells forming in the first place, does act in the same way as a vaccine for those who already have cancer cells proliferating in their bodies. The effect is not just the elimination of cancer at the ablation site, but also the stimulation of a complete response against all of that cancer cell type in the body. Essentially, the patient's own tumor has created a vaccine response in the body. Different than most vaccines, a vaccine made from your own tumor in your body is specific for you. It may also target numerous tumor antigens, giving the immune system antigen diversity. This way even if a cancer tries to hide, by mutating and disguising an antigen, this technique of *AblationVax™* can have multiple targets, so the cancer typically would have to hide numerous antigens at once, which is far less likely to happen. This diversity contrast is different from, and superior to, typical "off the shelf" cancer vaccines or therapies such as original CAR-T, which only target one antigen. It is the difference between just having a photo of a criminal suspect, versus having a photo, finger prints, DNA, height, weight, scars/tattoos. The more identifying aspects you have on your suspect, the better chances you can locate them. And it may take more than just a change in hairstyle or growing a mustache to avoid being captured. The tumor may need to do more than hiding a few antigens, which is certainly a common escape mechanism for cancer to evade the immune system.

This technique has shown a great initial response in cancer patients, and we are adding new combinations of agents almost monthly. I have no doubt that ablation with the right combination of immune agents could cure cancer in a high percentage of patients. But the important point is that you understand that immunotherapy by itself, or ablation by itself, are not nearly as effective as the combination of the two together. There is no comparison. Just because a patient has failed immunotherapy alone, or cryoablation alone, does not mean they cannot still be saved. If immune checkpoint inhibitors are removing the "brakes" of the immune system, then ablation is stomping on the gas pedal. To achieve the best outcome, both procedures must be done simultaneously. Only then can the patient's immune system get started in the right direction. I will add that as new combinations of immunotherapy are developed, maybe the ablation will become less necessary for stimulating the immune response.

In the next chapter, you will learn more about some new exciting combinations of immunotherapy agents injected into the tumor, which is taking immunotherapy to a whole new level.

CHAPTER 5

Intra-tumoral Immunotherapy "The Cure is Within You"

T HE CURE FOR cancer is within you. There is no better location for the immune system to learn to attack a cancer than within the tumor itself. These new immunotherapy drugs can have powerful effects, but they need to be in the right location. There have been numerous animal studies and some limited human work with injection of some of the FDA-approved immune checkpoint inhibitors, like anti-CTLA-4 and anti-PD-1, that certainly are very promising. However, the research world is beginning to move past these into some newer areas that look even more exciting.

In late January of 2018 a study was published by researchers at Stanford looking at the intra-tumoral injection (directly into the cancer) of the immunotherapy agent OX40 agonist antibody, combined with a Toll-like receptor agonist.

The results were astounding, with cures in all the mice. This led to some very huge news coverage and has set into motion exciting work in humans. We personally are already studying this and similar variations. Systemic treatments with immune checkpoint inhibitors like Opdivo, Keytruda and Yervoy were just the opening act. Now intra-tumoral injection with these other agents is primed to be the closer. There are far too many of these agents to discuss, so I am going to keep this discussion to the ones that I feel are the most important and that have almost immediate clinical relevance.

OX40 Agonist

OX40 receptor, also called CD134, is part of the tumor necrosis factor receptor super family. This is a co-stimulatory molecule and is expressed on activated T and antigen presenting cells. This receptor is the opposite of many of the other immunotherapy agents we have described that are widespread in current treatments today, such as anti-PD-1 and anti-CTLA-4. As described, those agents block receptors that are the brakes of the immune system. OX40 would be more equivalent to the gas pedal. OX40 actually has a dual function; it can remove the brakes (regulatory cells) and also increase T cell activation (stepping on the gas). Unlike the therapies for the traditional immune checkpoint inhibitors used today, with OX40 we are not blocking the receptor. We are activating it. As commonly found with most of these immune receptors, you will find these in many locations and they can function differently based on where they are located. In this case, the OX40 agonist (stimulating) antibody works in two ways. It stimulates the immune activation, but also binds to regulatory (inhibiting) cells and results in their destruction. The simple way to describe it is that OX40 agonist removes the brake and steps on the gas at the same time.

As mentioned, the Stanford study created significant media attention. This study points out several key points, one being that for good success, combinations are going to be needed. In this case, it was a Toll-like receptor (TLR) agonist with an OX40 agonist. Another key point is that intra-tumoral (injection into the tumor) is also essential, as some of these medications cannot be delivered to the entire body without potentially catastrophic consequences. This has one other advantage: the reduced doses will also reduce the cost. This is very important as we are already seeing that with current treatment methods the healthcare system cannot support the cost. Ultimately patients are missing out on their chance at these life-saving medications.

We are currently treating human patients of multiple cancer types with OX40/CpG agonist injected into the tumor, like the Stanford mouse study. The results have been extremely impressive. We have found that for humans, to get even better results, we have had to add the CTLA-4 inhibitor Yervoy. We plan to present and publish our initial results this year (2019).

Toll-Like Receptor Agonist

Toll-like receptors (TLR) are proteins that can recognize various non-specific pathogenic and dangerous substances. As mentioned, immune responses in cells such as T cells are very focused, recognizing very specific aspects of the cells and pathogens that they attack. That type of response must be stimulated and developed. TLR is part of the initial immune response, known as the innate immune system. When a new pathogen, or in our case, cancer is recognized, the immune system will not have a specific target and needs to recognize general aspects that may be associated with things believed to be dangerous. Then, with the right stimulus, these can convert to a more effective and specific immune response. The best way to understand this is going back to our car analogy. If the other immune agents we discussed are removing the brake and stepping on the gas, TLR are turning the key and cranking the car. As you can imagine, if the car is not running, removing the brake and stepping on the gas will have no effect. This is what can lead to failure of the traditional immunotherapy agents. They forget to crank the car. Also, in immunotherapy, it is not only the right combination of agents, but the correct sequence as well, that is vital for success. There are some studies showing that immunotherapy in the wrong order may negatively affect your future potential for a successful immune response. First you need to stimulate the immune system to be attracted to the tumor. A good example goes back to the Stanford Cancer Vaccine study, in which the researchers used the TLR to get the immune response started, then ramped it up and further activated it with the OX40 agonist. As you can see, one without the other and your car is not likely to go anywhere. It was this combination that proved to be highly effective in the study.

For an effective immune response, the immune system not only needs to recognize cancer, it needs to know that it is dangerous and should be eliminated. One key aspect to TLR agonists is that they will attract the immune response to the area they are located. This means that you cannot use the drugs systemically throughout the body such as oral or IV administration. These need to be used directly at a tumor site. As I have mentioned, most drug companies prefer systemic administration as it is easier to give, oncologists are not trained to inject tumors, and they are the ones that control most cancer treatment, and certainly drugs injected into tumors will generate less revenue than ones given systemically. There is an FDA-approved topical TLR agonist called Imiquimod, trade name Aldara. This is used in certain skin cancers and is being evaluated for topical use in breast cancer as well. In the Stanford study, they looked at the direct injection of a TLR 9 agonist, called CpG and a TLR 7/8 agonists called Resiquimod. CpG are short single strands of DNA that are found in high amounts in certain bacteria. The immune system has evolved to recognize these as being dangerous, which helps activate an immune response. This is considered the main active component in Coley's toxins, which were killed bacteria that Dr. Coley injected into cancers to help stimulate an immune response against cancer over 100 years ago. Think of CpG being the more refined version. This is an important aspect of generating an immune response. However, in most cases, it was not enough to do it alone. There was something missing to take the immune response to the next level. Ultimately there may prove to be several immune agents capable of advancing the initial immune response of TLR agonist to a durable cancer cure. OX40 agonist looks like it could be one of those missing pieces, at least in some cancers.

In the war against cancer, one important and forgotten aspect is getting your troops to the right location. If there are no troops, then activating them will do no good. This is one of the main reasons traditional immunotherapy may not work: The tumor environment does not have enough immune cells present. When immune cells are present, we call that an "inflamed or hot tumor environment," which has a better prognosis. When immune cells are not present, we call that an "immune desert or cold tumor environment," which has a poor prognosis. There needs to be signals to attract the immune cells to the tumor. However, this is even a little more complicated than you might think. The immune cells do not just swim to a tumor. The cells lining blood vessels must summon them. Since tumors control local vessel growth, you may guess that for tumors to survive and avoid the immune response, they build vessels that are less likely to attract the immune cells. They actually have vessels that may bring in regulatory cells to protect them and destroy the effector (attacker) T cells that want to kill them. Essentially, the tumor controls the roads in its territory, so it will keep out the enemy. This is another barrier to the immune system. A great review article published by Johansson-Percival, et al. in *Trends in Immunology;* "Immunomodulation of Tumor Vessels: It Takes Two to Tango" is an excellent overview of the current understanding of this process. One reason I mention this here is that it has been shown that CpG can help initiate changes in the vessels, which can then attract the needed immune cells. Think of the immune cells being on a train that can only get off where there is a stop. The cancer instructs blood vessels to form without stops for the attacking immune cells so they can't get off. Cpg helps make a stop so that immune cells now can get off where the tumor is located. As you can imagine, you can do everything possible to stimulate your immune system with the typical immunotherapy drugs, but if the immune cells never get to the tumor, the therapy cannot work.

This further supports the critical importance of intra-tumoral injection of CpG.

The other agent they mention in the article that can help, is low dose anti-VEGF drug, bevacizumab (Avastin), which we will talk more about later in this book.

STING Agonist

Stimulator of interferon genes (STING) is a protein that recognizes foreign pieces of nucleic acids (DNA/RNA) often found in cells that are infected with pathogens such as viruses. The recognition of these foreign nucleic acids triggers an innate immune response with secretion of immune-stimulating cytokines, such as interferon. This has a lot of similarities to the previously mentioned TLR agonist and overlaps with Coley's toxins as well. These STING agonists set up an initial immune response which can ultimately prime the T cells to be ready. As mentioned, it is the T cell response that leads to a more specific and durable anti-cancer immune response. The T cells are the main target of the currently approved immunotherapies such as anti-PD-1 and anti-CTLA-4. Again, if the T cells are not recruited and stimulated in the local cancer microenvironment, then these popular approved immunotherapies are unlikely to be effective. It is for this reason that agents stimulating an initial innate immune response such as TLR and STING agonist are gaining a lot of attention. In cases where the initial immune response is absent, to use current immune checkpoint inhibitors is essentially putting the cart before the horse. In addition, as I mentioned with the TLR agonist CpG, it seems that STING agonist can also cause changes to the vascular structures which enhance tracking of the immune cells back into the tumor environment. It also creates those new "train stops" for the T attackers.

Glen Barber, PhD, from the University of Miami, discovered STING in 2008 when he showed that mice lacking STING were very prone to viral infections. Later, Russell Vance, PhD, from UC Berkeley published in *Nature* 2011 that cyclic diguanylate monophosphate found in bacteria activates STING and stimulates an initial innate immune response. Basically, as later discovered by Zhijian Chen, of the University of Texas, Southwestern, there is an enzyme that links these nucleic acid pieces into a circle and that stimulates STING. Normally our own DNA would be located in the nucleus and would not trigger this response. This has now led to the development of synthetic cyclic dinucleotide (CDN) or other small molecules to activate STING. There have also been animal studies showing that the combination of TLR and STING agonist seem to work together, further enhancing the anti-cancer immune response. Certainly the STING agonist may have a bright future in cancer immunotherapy, but currently it is not as developed as the TLR agonist. Even though the drug companies hope to develop a STING agonist that can be given systemically, most of the initial work shows the promise is with intra-tumoral injection. I suspect the real benefits will come with combining both the TLR and STING agonist, injected directly into the tumor, still with other immune agents such as OX40 agonist.

One thing to note with STING agonist is that there are human and mouse versions of STING. Researchers were studying a STING agonist in mice called DMXAA. It looked extremely successful, but did poorly in human trials. This allowed them to realize that some substances, such as

DMXAA, may only bind to the mouse STING. The synthetic cyclic nucleotides (CDN) that were first studied activate STING in both humans and mice. However, researchers have been trying to find other small molecules that may be given in a different method than just injecting into the tumor. I understand their reasoning, but intra-tumoral injection will continue to be the safest and most effective route of administration of drugs such as STING and TLR agonist. In addition, researchers from Tufts University, Larkin, et al. (*J. Immunol.* 2017, DOI:10.4049) showed that high doses of STING agonist can have the opposite than desired effect and cause T cell death. So, as you can imagine, it will be hard to create a pill or IV therapy that would not give someone too much of the drug, since you must flood the body just to get enough in the locations of the tumor. This further supports that case that intra-tumoral administration should be superior.

As I was writing this book, a publication by Zhang, et al., "Identification of α-Mangostin as an Agonist of Human STING" was released in October 2018. This is an exciting development. They also described that mangostin may help convert tumor-protecting macrophages into tumor-attacking ones, another key area of immune resistance. It is interesting as mangostin comes from the fruit of the mangosteen tree (not to be confused with mangos). It is nice to know that this potentially very important cancer medication can be derived from a natural fruit. It is unclear if just eating the fruit would have much benefit or not. If it does, I suspect it would be for a different reason than the STING agonist.

A 2014 thesis by Dr. Fabiola Gutierrez Orozco, Ohio State University, indicated that mangostin extracts ingested orally may have a negative effect on the microbiome, increasing inflammation and reducing bacterial diversity. This makes sense, as it is to be expected that it would create a direct inflammatory response, attracting the immune cells. This is something you want in your tumor, but not necessarily in other areas of your body, like the colon. Further supporting the direct injection approach.

Intra-tumoral injection of vaccines, viruses and vaccine adjuvants

There are numerous techniques to stimulate an immune response into a tumor. It has been noted that in certain cases vaccines intended to prevent other illness may inadvertently stimulate an immune response within cancer. Myers, et al. published in March 2005 an article "Oncolytic activities of approved mumps and measles vaccines for therapy of ovarian cancer." They state: "In this study we demonstrated that two commercially available paramyxoviral vaccines, Moraten measles and Jeryl Lynn mumps have promising anti-tumor activities against human ovarian xenografts established in the peritoneal cavities of immunodeficient mice." Galanis, et al., also from Mayo, published January 2015 in *Cancer Res* that the use of the Edmonston vaccine strain of the measles virus showed effectiveness in the treatment of ovarian cancer, in patients who had previously received extensive chemotherapy, extending survival to 26.5 months in a group of 16 patients. Msaouel, et al., also from Mayo, reported anti-tumor activity with the same Edmonston measles vaccine. I might add that this is the old version of the measles vaccine.

Curiously, about the time of some of these publications, these vaccines have become hard to find, and it seems their sale in the U.S. has been blocked, as now everything has shifted to the use of the MMR in place of the older vaccine. I won't speculate the coincidence of the timing of this. As you see from the study, the results are not perfect, but I am sure the success can be increased with the combined use of other immunotherapy agents.

In July of 2018, Mckenzie and Nichols published in *JAMA Dermatology* a study in which a 97-year old woman with squamous cell carcinoma of the skin was treated successfully with a series of injections of Gardasil, the HPV vaccine. They initially injected the patient in the arm, to initiate an immune reaction, and then followed up with injection into the tumor. They noted that non-treated lesions resolved as well. There are numerous viruses or viral-based gene therapies that can be injected into tumor and can stimulate an immune response. Like most treatments, the use of these alone is probably not enough to generate a cure in most patients, but this can probably be significantly improved when used with the right combination of immunotherapy agents.

It is also reasonable to mention that, just like in vaccines, for the combination of immunotherapy agents to be effective, they often need a carrier agent, known as a vaccine adjuvant. This can be a key aspect to generating an immune response. In our work, we use Montanide ISA 51 or Saponin-based vaccine adjuvants, sometimes with a gel delivery. The idea is not only to enhance antigen delivery to the immune cells, but also to create a slow release formulation, keeping the medicines in the tumor environment. Montanide ISA 51 is used in several vaccines as an adjuvant because it is a water and oil-based mixture that enhances antigen delivery. It seems that the oil can solubilize some of the medications and create a slow release delivery system.

Another promising intra-tumoral therapy involves the use of a gene therapy that causes the increased production of Interleukin 12 within the tumor. IL-12 can activate both natural killer cells (NK) and attacking (cytotoxic) T cells. Studies are being done to inject the gene in a plasmid within the tumor. In addition, the gene can be placed within a virus and injected into the tumor. In this case, both the virus itself and the increase in production of IL-12 can stimulate an immune response against the cancer.

In addition, there are a few other immunotherapy agents that are being studied which all have excellent potential, alone or better yet in combination with other previously described agents. These are the ones I am particularly interested in: CD27, CD40 and CD137 (4-1BB) agonists. We are currently working with these and looking at the combinations with other immunotherapy agents. Like I said, we have most of the weapons needed, we just need to learn more about the right combinations.

As you can see from this chapter there are numerous therapies that can be injected directly into the tumor to stimulate an immune response. These combined with some of the other traditional immunotherapies, such as immune checkpoint inhibitors, may hold the key to highly effective cancer cures. In addition, because they are directly injected, they can reduce the number of needed treatments, side effects, and overall cost of therapy, which is a win all the way around.

CHAPTER 6

Other Important Immunotherapy Targets and Therapies

Transforming Growth Factor- Beta (TGF-B)

TGF-B IS AN important cytokine in regards to the immune response. Basically it inhibits the cancer attacking cells of the immune system and turns them into cancer protecting regulatory cells. TGF-B is also involved in the migration of cancer cells to new locations in the body. TGF-B may not only be produced by the cancer, but also is produced in the tissue surrounding the cancer (stroma). TGF-B both suppresses the immune response and increases migration, and also stimulates other growth factors, such as VEGF, to increase the blood vessels for cancer and make it more aggressive. In our previous discussions, I have mentioned that you can have different degrees of immune infiltration of cancer, the so-called "hot" versus "cold" tumor. We know that tumors that do not have immune cell infiltration or "cold," are not as likely to respond to immunotherapy. In an article published by Ros, May 2018, *Trends Cancer*, they describe how blocking TGF-B may be a key aspect in changing a "cold" tumor to a "hot" one. But there are some aspects of TGF-B that may be beneficial, so eliminating it completely may not be the best answer. There are drugs currently being tested which block more specific aspects, like the receptors, which should provide an anti-cancer response while not reducing the benefits TGF-B may provide. In an article published April 2018 in *Immunity,* Ganesh showed that combining immune checkpoint inhibitors with TGF-B inhibition induced a complete resolution of cancer in the mouse model.

There are still further studies needed, but there is some suggestion that the act of surgery, biopsies, ablation and radiation may increase TGF-B, further adding to immune suppression. In our work, we are looking at techniques to minimize this in respect to ablation. Also, considering the overall importance of TGF-B in the immune response, TGF-B receptor inhibitors are probably going to prove to be an invaluable weapon in cancer immunotherapy. This is an area we are actively studying as well.

TGF-B can be measured in the blood, which means it can be a helpful marker. In a study published by Sheng-Shin Wang, *Cryobiology,* May 2016, they describe how TGF-B levels can be useful in monitoring pre- and post treatment and when increases in the level occur after cryoablation of prostate cancer, they were more likely to have recurrence. We are now making it standard in our practice to get serial TGF-B levels to evaluate treatment options and potential results.

While commercially available and FDA-approved TGF-B inhibitors may be a few years away, there are reported to be a few natural inhibitors of TGF-B. Although there still needs to be further studies in this area, I recommend to my patients Berberine, Curcumin, Capsaicin, EGCG, Selenium and Sulforaphane. There must be caution with EGCG, since in rare cases, high doses can cause liver damage. I also think Black Cumin Seed oil is a good option and we regularly use Losartan.

Here is a limited listed of a few natural TGF-B inhibitors that appear in medical literature:

1. Curcumin, reported by Thacker, *PLoS One*, March 2016.

2. Capsaicin (component of chili peppers) reported by Choi, et al. *J Agric Food Chem*; Jan 2018.

3. Epicatechin-3-gallate (EGCG) Green Tea, reported by Huang, SF, et al.; *Food Chem Toxicol.* Aug 2016.

4. Sulforaphane (Broccoli Seed Extract), reported by Wu, J, et al., *Oncol Rep.* May 2016.

5. Berberine (plant extract, barberry) reported by Kim, et al. "Berberine Suppresses Cell Motility Through Downregulation of TGF-B1 in Triple Negative Breast Cancer Cells" *Cellular Physiology and Biochemistry* 2018; 45:795-807.

6. Selenium, Lennicke, et al.; Poster presentation SITC 2017, "Selenium, the element of the moon improves immunotherapy on earth."

Also of possible interest:

7. Red Ginseng Oil, report by Truong in *Molecules*, Sept 2017.

8. Black Cumin Seed Oil (Thymoquinone) Mostofa, et al. "Thymoquinone as a Potential Adjuvant Therapy for Cancer Treatment: Evidence from Preclinical Studies." *Frontiers in Pharmacology,* June 2017.

Off-label drugs that inhibit TGF-B include:

9. Losartan reported by Arnold "Losartan Slows Pancreatic Tumor Progression and Extends Survival of SPARC-Null Mice by Abrogating Aberrant TGF-B Activation." *PLoS One*, Feb 14, 2012.

CSF1R

As we have discussed, the immune cells in the tumor microenvironment play a key role in dictating the cancer immune response, for good or bad. Most of the current approved immunotherapies focus on the T cell, which in cancer immunotherapy, though important, is very one-dimensional. There are other cells in the microenvironment that play a huge role in the suppression of the immune system in cancer, specifically tumor-associated macrophages (TAMs) and myeloid-derived suppressor cells (MDSCs). As mentioned before, your immune system has two sides, one that attacks cancer and the other that protects it. TAMs and MDSCs protect it. To enhance our immune response we want to eliminate, deactivate, or change TAMs and MDSCs. It is now recognized that one area of weakness of the currently approved immunotherapy options is that they do not address

TAMs or MDSCs. This is where blocking colony-stimulating factor 1 receptor (CSF1R) is going to play an essential role. By blocking the CSF1R it can reprogram some of these cancer protecting immune cells into cancer attacking ones. Blocking CSF1R also increases PD-L1 and CTLA-4, making the immune system more responsive to these typical immune checkpoint inhibitors, further supporting the need for a combination therapy. Though I do not like to generalize the immunotherapy response potential (immunogenicity) of any particular tumor type, some studies suggest that CSF1R blockade may be more important in pancreatic and prostate cancers. I suspect in the future we will look at CSF1/CSF1R on a personalized level to identify the specific patients this therapy is likely to benefit the most.

Tumor Infiltrating Lymphocytes (TILs)

In the tumor microenvironment there may be present T cells that are recognizing the cancer and trying to fight it. The concept behind TILs is, if possible, harvest cells that want to attack the cancer. If you stimulate these cells and grow more outside the body, then re-infuse them to the patient, they may be powerful enough to eliminate the cancer. It is a reasonable concept that is already showing some success. This technique is gaining more attention now because of research published by Dr. Steven Rosenberg in *Nature Medicine*, June 2018, demonstrating complete regression in an advanced breast cancer patient using this technique. They selected out TILs that reacted against 4 different mutant proteins of the cancer, growing those and infusing them into the patient. This therapy, though promising, still has some drawbacks. One is that you have to deplete the patient's immune system with chemotherapy; the other is that this technique is extremely expensive. I do not want to downplay too much the benefits of this type of therapy, but it is still my belief that intra-tumoral immunotherapy has better potential, both in terms of success and practicality.

Chimeric Antigen Receptor T Cells (CAR-T)

CAR-T is getting a lot of attention, mainly in blood born cancers. There are two FDA-approved CAR-T, one for diffuse large B cell lymphoma, the other for relapsed/refractory B cell precursor acute lymphoblastic leukemia. The idea with CAR-T is that you genetically engineer the T cell to express an antibody receptor that targets a receptor on the cancerous cells. This has proven to be effective in blood cancer that has specific targets, but not so easy in the majority of cancers, which are of the solid type. In most solid cancers, it would not be enough to target just one mutation because cancer can generally outsmart one-dimensional treatments targeting one mutation by hiding the expression of that protein. In addition, CAR-T has been plagued with side effects issues, such as cytokine release syndrome (CRS). However, in Chapter 11, I discuss how this may now not be as much of a problem with the use of an IL-1 blocking drug in combination with CAR-T. Certainly as the technology improves, there is a good future with these drugs, and at the moment they are gaining a lot of attention from the media and investors, but their transition to clinical use in patients has been more challenging. The huge price tag they come with does not help either.

CHAPTER 7

The Effect of Traditional Cancer Treatments On the Cancer Immune Response—The Good, The Bad and The Ugly

C LEARLY I THINK every cancer patient knows their basic traditional options for cancer treatment. If cancer is caught early, it is often surgery, probably with chemotherapy and radiation to follow, that is typically prescribed. If cancer is caught late, or if the patient was treated early, but the cancer has nonetheless progressed, treatment options generally are going to center around chemotherapy, radiation, and maybe the combination of both. I am a traditionally trained doctor, but I am not a fan of these treatment options. I have seen the results first-hand and in general, they are pretty disappointing.

Patients would like a more effective therapy, hopefully with fewer side effects. Our main goal is to eliminate these treatments that seem rather barbaric. More and more, patients are questioning the logic of these treatments, instead of following their doctor's recommendation blindly. The cancer system is very hesitant to get away from these therapies. Immunotherapy has come on the scene and is becoming accepted at a fast pace, and its acceptance in large part is patient driven. Patients see the ads, hear the success stories, and question their doctor about getting immunotherapy. Still in most cases, even though the results with immunotherapy are better, it is often held back until oncologists can get a few courses of chemo and radiation in first. To me, this is like saying, "Yes we have something that works better, but let's try the stuff that doesn't work well first, and then later we can try something that might work better. Oh, and we are going to beat up your body first, so that later your chances of immunotherapy working will be even less."

This clearly makes no sense. The healthcare industry is addicted to chemotherapy and radiation just like the energy industry is addicted to oil. It is for this reason that the system is slow to change. I have to admit, to completely abandon the current treatments is something that would create an economic crisis, and for that reason the changes will be gradual. That being said, the immunotherapy industry is going to be big business in its own right. Big Pharma is already getting themselves well entrenched as the change is coming, though the hospitals and the doctors are still lagging behind.

However, enough on those aspects, our goal here is to give you the information to enhance your treatment success. So, can chemotherapy and radiation be used to your advantage?

Yes it can. Could it be that chemotherapy and radiation may be detrimental to immunotherapy treatments? Yes to that also. There is still a lot for us to understand about the interaction of these traditional treatments and immunotherapy. I will try to guide you to make the most out of these combinations. The reality is that most cancer patients, if they stay inside the standard healthcare system, whether it is for convenience or insurance coverage, are probably going to get chemotherapy. Let's make the most out of it.

Chemotherapy and the Immune Response

In general, it has been recognized that chemotherapy will suppress the immune system. Certainly decreased white blood counts are a common issue with chemotherapy. However, even in the face of decreasing the white blood cells counts, chemotherapy can have immune-stimulating aspects. This certainly seems like a contradiction until we remember that the immune system has two faces, one that attacks tumors and one that protects them. So, if you can weaken the protecting side (regulatory cells that include Tregs and MDSCs) more, then you can end up with a net positive in the overall anti-cancer immune response. In addition, killing cancer is like reducing its troops, making it more susceptible. It is like a war, you can have death on both sides that are fighting, but if there is more death on the opposing side, you are winning.

So, what are some of the effects that chemotherapy can have that are beneficial? One is immunogenic tumor cell death by mechanisms that cause a release of tumor antigens and stimulate danger signals. Tumors dying by these methods can help enhance an immune response. In addition, cancer as it is growing produces many immune-inhibiting substances, both by direct protein production and byproducts of its own metabolism. If you directly suppress cancer growth with chemotherapy, you can reduce these, making the job for the immune system easier. There are certain chemotherapy agents that may be associated with increasing the immune response. I will address these directly. This being said, if you are going to get treated with chemotherapy and you have an option of different drugs, you may want to keep in mind ones that can have a more positive effect on the immune response. Also, if you are going to get chemotherapy, you really need to try to take advantage of the potential synergy with immunotherapy. I know this is easier said than done, as most oncologists have not gotten on board with this combination therapy. In addition, low and frequently dosed chemotherapy, called metronomic dosing, seems to be superior when it comes to stimulating an immune response. Sadly, this is not how oncologists usually administer chemotherapy. "A Combination of Immune Checkpoint Inhibition with Metronomic Chemotherapy as a Way of Targeting Therapy-Resistant Cancer Cells," an article published in the *International Journal of Molecular Sciences*, Oct 13, 2017 discussed how metronomic chemotherapy can reduce tumor growth, which reduces immune-suppressing metabolic byproducts, such as lactic acid. It can also decrease tumor angiogenesis, regulatory immune cells, and also inhibit the tissue stroma that may actually be supporting the cancer. As much as we all would like to see chemotherapy become a distant memory, it still can have its uses, especially in the current immunotherapy situation. If the patient has very bulky, advanced cancer, they may need the help of some chemotherapy to get it more under control for the immune system to have a fighting chance. Otherwise, an advanced and rapid growing cancer can actually outpace the immune system. The cancer has usually had a significant head start, so chemo may slow it down, allowing the immune system to catch up.

I want to stress that if chemotherapy is what you need, you should strongly look into the low dose metronomic chemotherapy since it can achieve many of the goals of slowing cancer, and may boost the anti-cancer immune response.

What follows is a look at some of the most commonly used chemotherapy drugs.

Gemcitabine

Gemcitabine has been shown to cause tumor cell death that stimulates an immune response. It also can decrease regulatory cells, such as Tregs and MDSCs. An article published by Zhao, et al. (*Immunology Lett.* 2017 Jan; 181:36-44), demonstrated that Gemcitabine could decrease Tregs, reduce suppressive cytokines, such as TGF-B, and increase stimulatory cytokines like Interferon-gamma. This was in low dose therapy in mice. As mentioned, the immune-stimulating aspects of chemotherapy seem to occur when it is used with frequent low dosing (metronomic). This certainly requires further study, but this goes against the typical chemotherapy dosing scheme that uses a maximum tolerated dose therapy, which is intermittent, but high dosing.

5-Fluorouracil (5FU)

5FU also in a low dose fashion was shown in animal studies to enhance the immune response by increasing antigen presentation. However, Wu, et al. published in *BMC Immunology*, Sept. 20, 2016, research showing that repeated doses of 5FU impaired the anti-cancer immune response of T cells, as opposed to a single dose. Again, most studies are supporting that low dose or limited chemotherapy may enhance an immune response. The problem is getting an oncologist who is willing to give chemotherapy in this manner.

Cyclophosphamide

Low dose cyclophosphamide has also been shown to enhance an anti-cancer immune response. In a study published by Scurr, et al. in *Clinical Cancer Research*, Nov. 15, 2017, they showed that low dose cyclophosphamide induced an anti-tumor T cell response in metastatic colorectal cancer that was associated with increased survival. Levy, et al. from Johns Hopkins published in *The Journal of Pharmacology and Experimental Therapeutics* (330:596-601, 2009) that low dose cyclophosphamide unmasked the anti-metastatic effect of local tumor cryoablation. This study showed that cryoablation with cyclophosphamide, but not surgery, demonstrated a systemic anti-cancer immune response. In the animal model of metastatic colorectal cancer, survival rates achieved by using cyclophosphamide plus cryoablation was shown to be 50%, compared to 0% when combined with surgery or versus cryoablation alone. One common dosing regimen is to use 50mg by mouth every other day. This has little, if any toxicity and high ease of use, since it is in a pill form. We often use this regimen ourselves, especially when combined with cryoablation.

Doxorubicin

Doxorubicin is a chemotherapy agent that works by interfering with DNA replication. It originated from soil bacteria and is considered an anti-tumor antibiotic. It generally has a bad reputation for its side effects. Besides bone marrow suppression and hair loss, toxicity to the heart can be a major problem. It is red in color and often is called "Red Death." On the positive side, it does seem to have some immune-stimulating aspects by killing tumors in a manner that may attract the immune system. At this time there is not much data on the combination of Doxorubicin with immunotherapy, but as with other chemo drugs, we would expect a low dose to stimulate the immune response and have reduced side effects.

Radiation Therapy and the Effect on the Immune Response

Like certain aspects of chemotherapy and ablation, radiation will cause tumor killing, and the resultant dead pieces of tumor can act as antigens delivered to the immune system. In general, radiation therapy may be considered immunosuppressive, but when combined with immunotherapy there seems to be synergy. I will admit that I am biased, and I feel that cryoablation is superior to radiation in its ability to stimulate an immune response; however, it will be easier for the average patient to obtain radiation, than cryoablation. It is just a sheer numbers and insurance game; there is a lot more radiation therapy available than cryoablation. Insurance coverage for radiation is generally much easier to come by than for cryoablation. So, we might as well make use of what we have available.

If you are to get radiation, it would probably serve you well to also have immunotherapy. But even though there is good evidence for the combination, getting a doctor willing to actually do it is easier said than done. Again, cryoablation certainly would be my first choice, but let's explore radiation further.

One area we have not discussed much is something called MHC-I, which is expressed on the cell surface. The job of MHC-I is to present to immune cells internal peptides that may be foreign. Think of it almost like a distress signal. This is presented to the immune system so that it will know if it needs to destroy the cell or not. It is almost as if the immune system was searching for someone, and the cell presents its ID. If the ID matches the person it is looking for, in this case, cancer, then the cell is destroyed. In some cases, the cancer can escape by not having MHC on the surface. Think of it like the cancer having a fake ID. So the immune system gives it a pass. Radiation therapy can make cells that are hiding their MHC show it again. Radiation can also activate the stimulator of interferon genes (STING) pathway, which can stimulate a non-specific innate immune response. On the downside, it can cause the release of TGF-B and VEGF, which are both immune suppressive. Also, radiation can reduce white blood count, which is associated with immune suppression. There are numerous studies looking at the combination of radiation and immunotherapy. There are still some issues to be sorted out, such as determining what dose and how frequently radiation therapy should be administered. What is the timing of immunotherapy, before, after, during? There are some conflicting studies related to these treatment details. I suspect in the next couple of years these will get worked out. However, I hope in the next couple of years the need for radiation therapy will be significantly diminished as it is replaced with more effective treatments with less side effects. I might add that I have personally seen cases where patients were failing with immunotherapy, then when radiation was added the immune response kicked in. So there are some real potential benefits and certainly patients who are failing or have failed immunotherapy might want to consider adding in radiation to potentially activate the immune response.

As you have seen from this chapter, there may be some benefits to be gained from traditional older cancer treatments such as chemotherapy and radiation associated with an anti-cancer immune response. There are currently numerous studies underway. The one thing to consider when it comes to chemotherapy is that most studies are focused on the traditional delivery method of maximum tolerated dose chemotherapy, but the science points in the direction of a lower but more frequent dosing as being superior. There are doctors that offer a low dose, metronomic chemotherapy, but most are not your traditional oncologists, so you may have to do some searching.

In addition, for a patient with advanced bulky disease, chemotherapy and radiation may be useful to decrease the tumor burden, making it easier for your immune system to fight. There is still more to be learned about the timing of administration. For example, certain mouse studies have showed that cyclophosphamide given before chemotherapy such as Doxorubicin may stimulate an anti-cancer immune response, but the reverse actually suppresses the immune response. These types of findings can be variable, depending on the cancer type and location as well as the local tumor immune environment, all of which can greatly affect the responses. Though it is still being evaluated, I have seen at immunology meetings presentations discussing when maximum dose chemotherapy is used first it may reduce the potential success of immunotherapy when used later. This most likely is related to the long-term immune suppression. Make sure to discuss low dose metronomic chemotherapy with your doctor, and hopefully they will be willing to oblige. It may be a good idea to go armed with studies. One good review is by Wu, *Cancer Letters* (2018) 419:210-221; Immunogenic chemotherapy: Dose and schedule dependence and combination with immunotherapy. I wish you the best of luck in convincing them; it may not only help you, but many future patients as well.

CHAPTER 8

Genetic and Molecular Targeted Cancer Drugs and Immunotherapy, Don't Miss Your Chance For Synergy

B OTH GENETIC AND molecular targeted cancer drugs can work synergistically with immunotherapies to improve outcomes. There are still risks involved, however. In this chapter, I will introduce you to some of the most noteworthy of these drugs.

PARP Inhibitors

PARP inhibitor [poly (ADP-ribose) polymerase inhibitor] drugs make up a class of medications most typically used with breast and ovarian cancers with BRCA1, BRCA2 or PALB2 mutations. In addition, it then may have some effect in cancers in which the tumor suppressor PTEN gene is defective. PARP is a protein that repairs breaks in the DNA. When the ability to repair these DNA breaks are inhibited, it can lead to the death of the cells. Rapidly dividing cells, such as cancer cells, would be more sensitive to this than normal cells.

A study published in the journal *Cancer Immunology Research*, November 2015, by Higuchi, et al., "CTLA-4 Blockade Synergizes Therapeutically with PARP Inhibition in BRCA1-Deficient Ovarian Cancer" demonstrated that CTLA-4 inhibitors, but not PD-1/PD-L1 inhibitors, enhanced the anti-cancer immune response and survival in the mouse model. However, in a human study with 60 patients with ovarian cancer that was resistant to platinum therapy, 25% of the patients had a complete or partial response using the combination of the PARP inhibitor niraparib with the PD-1 inhibitor pembrolizumab (Keytruda). This was versus 5% with the PARP alone and 11% with Keytruda alone. Also of note, these patients did not have BRCA mutations, which will increase the potential of patients that can be treated with this combination.

Studies have shown that PARP inhibitors increase the expression of PD-L1, which can increase the effectiveness of PD-1/PD-L1 inhibitors (*Clinical Cancer Research*, Jiao, et al. Feb 2017, "PARP inhibitor upregulates PD-L1 expression and enhances cancer-associated immunosuppression"). Some of the early results with human clinical trials have shown modest increase in survival time, but overall the results are still fairly lacking. Since we know that in general, for systemic immunotherapy, a PD-1/CTLA-4 inhibitor combination (Yervoy/Opdivo or Yervoy/Keytruda) can be effective at times, those combinations of drugs with a PARP inhibitor should be somewhat promising, as well.

CDK4/6 Inhibitors

Cyclin-dependent kinases 4 & 6 inhibitor, Palbociclib (Ibrance), is FDA-approved for ER-positive and HER2-negative breast cancer. Cyclin-dependent kinases are regulators of cell cycle and cell division and are important for progression of some cancers. In a study published by Goel, et al. in *Nature*, August 2017, they demonstrate that inhibitors of CDK4/6 can promote anti-tumor immunity. One mechanism was by increasing retroviral elements within cancers that resulted in increased double-stranded RNA. This caused an increase in interferons and antigen presentation. In addition, CDK4/6 inhibitors decrease T regulatory cells. These effects result in an increase in the cytotoxic T cell response (attacking T cells). Other studies, such as "The CDK4/6 Inhibitor Abemaciclib Induces a T Cell Inflamed Tumor Microenvironment and Enhances the Efficacy of PD-L1 Checkpoint Blockage" by Schaer, et al., support the idea that a combination of CDK4/6 inhibitors with immunotherapy, such as PD-1/PD-L1 inhibitors, should have good synergy. The ability to convert a "cold" tumor to a "hot/inflamed" one is a very key area that is lacking in traditional immune checkpoint therapy, leading to failure. Though the human data is still lacking, patients who are getting CDK4/6 inhibitors, should certainly look into the option of getting immunotherapy at the same time.

EGFR Inhibitors

EGFR inhibitors block the epidermal growth factor receptor, which is found on the surface of some cells stimulating cell growth. There are several types of EGFR inhibitors. They can be tyrosine kinase inhibitors or monoclonal antibodies. These are used in colon, breast, lung, pancreatic, renal and head and neck cancers. Although there have been very limited studies with the combination of EGFR inhibitors and immunotherapy, theoretically, the combination should be synergistic. However, in limited studies of patients who received PD-1 inhibitors combined with a TKI EGFR inhibitor a significant increase in side effects with modest increase in survival was observed. It is unclear what synergy may surface with other immunotherapies in the future. In addition, Schoenfeld, et al. published an article titled "Severe Immune Related Adverse Events Are Common with Sequential PD-(L)1 Blockade and Osimertinib" in *Annals of Oncology*, March 7, 2019. This article cites a human study which showed that patients first placed on a PD-1 or PD-L1 inhibitor, followed by the EGFR inhibitor osimertinib (Tagrisso), had increased adverse immune side effects. This was greatest if the drugs were started less than 3 months apart. The duration of use of the PD-1/PD-L1 inhibitor did not seem to matter. Of note, if the EGFR inhibitor was used first, no significant immune side effects were seen. Again, systemic use of these drugs, even when not done at the same time, can result in increased side effects. This begs the question, how would systemic EGFR receptor inhibitors work with intra-tumoral injection of PD-1/PD-L1 inhibitors?

Estrogen inhibitors

Estrogen inhibiting drugs are commonly used in estrogen receptor positive breast cancers. These include Tamoxifen, Fulvestrant, Letrozole and Anastrozole. In an article published by Svoronos, et al. in the journal *Cancer Discovery*, January 2017, titled "Tumor Cell-Independent Estrogen Signaling Drives Disease Progression Through Mobilization of Myeloid-Derived Suppressor Cells" they describe how estrogen inhibits anti-cancer immunity irrespective of the receptor status of the cancer. It is known that there are inherent differences in the immune systems of men and women, particularly related to hormonal differences. Estrogen receptors are not only expressed on some tumors, but are also expressed on immune cells. Studies are indicating that estrogen causes an increase in regulatory cells, such as MDSCs, along with reducing infiltration of CD8 positive, tumor-attacking T cells in the tumor microenvironment. The basic idea is that estrogen inhibiting drugs seem to have positive effects on the anti-cancer immune response, no matter if the cancer cells are estrogen receptor positive or not.

VEGF inhibitors

In February, 2019, Motzer, et al. published in the *New England Journal of Medicine* results of a human study with the combination of Avelumab (PD-L1 inhibitor) with Axitinib (INLYTA, a TKI inhibiting VEGF, C-Kit and PDGFR). This study showed that the combination extended progression-free survival by an additional 5.4 months over standard of care sunitinib (8.4 months to 13.8 months). I know that is modest, and I would certainly hope for better, but since Axitinib is a pill, it may be easy to add for patients who are having to stick more to standard of care immunotherapy.

One of the classic VEGF inhibitors is the monoclonal antibody drug, Bevacizumab (Avastin). In the clinical trial called IMpower 150, they studied 1200 advanced non-small cell lung cancer patients. The results showed that at one year the survival of the combination Bevacizumab with the PD-L1 inhibitor Atezolizumab (Tecentriq) was 37% versus 18% for Bevacizumab plus chemotherapy. In addition, they noted that patients with gene mutations had a similar response, when normally it was thought those patients did not have much benefit from immunotherapy.

VEGF is mainly known for its effect on angiogenesis, enhancing blood vessel growth to tumors. However, VEGF also causes immunosuppression in the tumor microenvironment. One aspect as mentioned before is that immune cells do not just swim to the tumor; they must be attracted to the area by the cells lining blood vessel walls. Excess VEGF in the tumor microenvironment leads to vessel formation that impedes the ability of immune cells to enter. Essentially, it helps create a barrier to the immune system. In addition, VEGF causes the increase of regulatory (tumor-protecting) immune cells, such as MDSCs and Tregs. Also, VEGF inhibits the maturation of dendritic cells. Mature dendritic cells present antigens to the other immune cells and stimulate an immune response, while immature dendritic cells function as regulatory cells, inhibiting an immune response. For all of these reasons, it makes sense that anti-VEGF drugs not only are effective against tumor vessel development, but also are actually immunotherapy agents in their own right. There are numerous anti-VEGF drugs that have FDA approval, besides the ones mentioned. Others currently in trials combined with immunotherapy include: Ramucirumab (CYRAMZA) and Nintedanib (Vargatef, Ofev).

CCR5 Inhibitor (Maraviroc)

Different than some of the other agents listed in this chapter, this is not only a targeted agent, but is also and "off-label" medication as well. Maraviroc is actually an FDA-approved anti-viral agent used for the treatment of HIV. This medication received FDA approval back in August 2007. Besides allergic and skin reactions, this drug does have liver toxicity, so liver function needs to be closely monitored. An article published by Aldinucci and Casagrande in the journal *International Journal of Molecular Sciences*, May 2018, titled "Inhibition of the CCL5/CCR5 Axis Against the Progression of Gastric Cancer" gives a great explanation of the underlying mechanism.

To give you a brief explanation, CCL5 binds to CCR5, causing the activation of the receptor. The activated receptor has multiple mechanisms of cancer stimulation. First, it causes direct proliferation of the cancer through mTOR, cyclin D1, C-Myc and Dad-1, along with increasing glucose metabolism. Second, it causes direct immunosuppression by recruiting regulatory immune cells, especially TAMs, that ultimately lead to the increase in inhibitory cytokines such as IDO, TGF-B and IL-10. Halama, et al. demonstrated that blocking CCR5 with Maraviroc led to converting tumor-associated macrophages (TAMs) from the M2 (tumor-protecting) to the M1 (tumor-attacking) type. Besides TAMs, it also seems that Maraviroc reprograms MDSCs as well. If that was not enough, Maraviroc also inhibits VEGF, tumor migration and metastasis formation.

MEK inhibitors

In 2016 results were presented at the European Society for Medical Oncology (ESMO) by Johanna Bendell, MD on a phase 1 study combining atezolizumab (PD-L1 inhibitor) with cobimetinib (MEK inhibitor) for patients with microsatellite stable (MSS) metastatic colorectal cancer. In general, MSS patients do not respond as well to immunotherapy and unfortunately make up the majority of patients (95%). This combination offers the hope that MSS metastatic colorectal patients may have an improved chance to respond to one of the most widely used type of immunotherapy, PD-1/PD-L1 inhibitors. The results were pretty modest, with 17% partial response, 22% stable disease, with a response duration from 4 months to greater than 15 months. The exact mechanism still seems to not be well understood, but most likely involves a decrease in immune suppressive mediators such as COX-2 and Arg1 with increasing cytotoxic T cell infiltration in the tumor microenvironment. Ebert el al published a study in *Immunity,* 2016 that MEK inhibition reduces CD8+ T cell apoptosis during chronic T cell receptor stimulation. Often when the immune system is chronically activated, like in cancer, the immune cells that attack the cancer can be fatigued and may die off. This indicates a MEK inhibitor may assist in preventing this immune suppression from developing. Certainly in patients who have MSS colorectal cancer and are considering systemic immunotherapy with a PD-1/PD-L1 inhibitor, this combination with a MEK inhibitor should be an option.

ALK inhibitors

Combinations can also be associated with problems. In an article published by Patel, et al. in *Journal of Thoracic Disease*, July 2018; titled "ALK Inhibitors and Checkpoint Blockade: A Cautionary Tale Mixing Oil with Water?" they describe the high incidence of hepatoxicity (liver toxicity) with this combination. In this study there were deaths due to the hepatotoxicity, leading to the trial being discontinued. There are a few things of note here. Even though PD-1/PD-L1 inhibitors have been considered a major advancement, they still have an overall low success rate and mild toxicity. In the future, I suspect this class of drugs will be replaced, or used as a follow up to other immunotherapies. In addition, toxicity from combinations that could be highly effective may be avoided by intra-tumoral injection.

CXCR4 Inhibitors (Plerixafor)

Cancer cells can have increased expression of CXCR4, which binds to CXCL12. This interaction can function as a homing mechanism for cancer. It also can increase fibrosis in the cancer tissues, which acts as a barrier from immune cells. In breast and lung cancer, patients with over-expression of CXCR4 have a worse prognosis. CXCR4 is also involved in other cancers, such as prostate, ovarian, colon and bladder. The drug Plerixafor is FDA-approved for the treatment of lymphoma and multiple myeloma. This allows for the off-label use in other cancers. In a study published in *PNAS*, Jan 30, 2019 by Chen, et al.; title "Blocking CXCR4 alleviates desmoplasia, increases T-lymphocyte infiltration, and improves immunotherapy in metastatic breast cancer" they describe how Perixafor enhances immune checkpoint therapy in the mouse model. This could lead to another target in immunotherapy. It is certainly possible to evaluate the patient's tumor for expression of CXCR4 to see if they may have potential benefit.

DDR2 Inhibitors

The most potent FDA-approved DDR2 inhibitor is Dasatinib (Sprycel), which is used in CML and ALL. It is a tyrosine kinase inhibitor, which besides DDR2, also targets BCR/Abl, Src, c-Kit and ephrin receptors. In a study published in Science Advances, Feb 20, 2019 by Tu, et al. title, "Targeting DDR2 enhances tumor response to anti-PD-1 immunotherapy" they describe the mechanisms of synergy in the mouse model. They describe that there is increased infiltration of CD8 positive T cells in both the tumor and spleen. This was unique to the combination. Though this is a limited study and human studies are needed, it does show promise that Dasatinib may enhance the effectiveness of PD-1 inhibitors, the most widely used type of immunotherapy at this time.

Still, there's more that can be done to empower the immune system to do its job, and this is where the patients themselves come in. There are some simple but novel steps that cancer patients can take to enhance the immune response. It's not just a gut feeling that I have that tells me cancer can be cured—it's the gut itself. Because believe it or not, what grows inside our guts can help our immune system save our lives. So turn the page and find out more.

CHAPTER 9

Gut Flora: The Key to Successful Immunotherapy

W HEN I HEAR of patients who have failed traditional immunotherapy, one of the first questions I ask myself is, did they have the right bacterial flora in their intestinal system? Were they eating a high fiber diet and taking the appropriate pre- and probiotics that they needed for their gut to enhance their immune system? Were they even aware of the connection between gut flora and the immune system? Chances are, they weren't.

I have to admit that when I first realized that the intestinal flora played a critical role in the function of immunotherapy, I was a bit shocked. Of course, I had known for years that many integrative doctors recommended probiotics, which are bacteria and yeasts that aid in the digestive process. I also knew that the gut is a major part of the immune system. But I hadn't appreciated the role of intestinal flora until the publication of two key studies showing that the appropriate bacteria in the intestines are critical for the function of today's current immune checkpoint inhibitors. Until then, I felt that these new immunotherapy drugs were so powerful that they stood on their own. I now know that intestinal bacteria is so crucial to effective immunotherapy that it can mean the difference between treatment success and failure.

To understand why, let's examine the evolution of our digestive systems. As our species has evolved, our guts have grown smaller. That is because early humans survived by eating a plant-based diet, which required a longer period—and more calories—to digest. Meat was scarce, and with no way to store it, when it was available it spoiled rapidly, so not much meat was consumed.

Human culture adapted to this diet by learning how to store foods that would otherwise spoil. Fermentation was one of the earliest forms of food storage, and appeared in diverse cultures throughout the world in the form of beer, wine, vinegars, and curdled milk products (such as cheeses which contained live molds and yogurts which contained living enzymes). Almost all cultures have some form of fermented vegetables, whether kimchee, sauerkraut, or other pickled vegetables. These foods all contained a rich biodiversity of living yeasts, bacteria and enzymes that were consumed and thrived in the gut and helped protect humans from disease. In other words, early humans learned to prepare and store foods in a manner that maintained a complex and diverse microbiology in their intestinal systems.

As we migrated northward, however, the cold environment limited plant production, but it enabled us to store and consume more meat. As our diets and environments changed, so did our bodies. The long gut necessary to digest a raw, plant-based diet was less necessary. As we ate more meat and cooked our foods, our guts grew smaller and more efficient in digestion. Shifting to a meat-based diet had its advantages—with less energy necessary to digest raw plant material, our brains developed more rapidly—but it also came with a major disadvantage. The biodiversity of our gut bacteria diminished, a process that has continued with changing technologies that have revolutionized our diets.

In our efforts to preserve foods for longer storage, and to kill harmful organisms present in foods, we have indiscriminately killed almost all the microorganisms present in our food. Preservation is now more likely to kill the healthy bacteria our bodies need, rather than maintain them. Pasteurization has done an amazing job of protecting us from food-borne diseases, but it has done so at the cost of killing the healthy bacteria along with the unhealthy organisms. Few foods we eat today contain the complex microbiology we once digested regularly. Our guts remain a critical defense system against disease, but the modern human gut has been weakened by our dietary and lifestyle changes.

One such change has been the widespread use of antibiotics—yet another example of how saving lives has come at a cost to human health. Let me explain.

When Louis Pasteur and Robert Koch introduced an early form of antibiotics in the late 19th century to treat *Bacillus anthracis*, bacteria present in livestock and humans (and from which the deadly pathogen anthrax was developed), it revolutionized medicine. The use of antibiotics became widespread in the mid-20th century and continued to be viewed as a miraculous drug—because they do save lives. But because antibiotics attack living bacteria, those bacteria that are resistant to antibiotics thrive over time through the process of natural selection. The result is that new forms of antibiotics must be continually developed in order to outwit the harmful bacteria, all the while other bacteria—many of which are healthy and essential to our immune systems—are destroyed.

Added to this antibiotic resistance is the contemporary practice of adding low doses of antibiotics to animal feed to ward off disease—antibiotics we digest in our meat-based diets. The result of all these dietary and food production changes is that our guts have changed—and not for the better. The modern guts of most people who subsist on a meat-based diet high in processed and refined foods have lost the diversity of microorganisms that our immune systems depend on to do their job.

Now let's turn to the role of antibiotics in cancer treatment. It is very common for cancer patients to receive antibiotic therapy sometime during their treatment, since their immune systems have been jeopardized and they develop various infections. In addition, some antibiotics are known to have anti-cancer properties in their own right. Though antibiotics are often necessary for treating infections, it is extremely important for them to be used appropriately. Studies are now indicating that treatment with antibiotics up to one-month prior starting immunotherapy may have negative effect. Pinato, et al. presented at the ASCO-SITC 2019 conference a poster of a multi-center trial looking at antibiotic use with PD-1/PD-L1 inhibitors. They showed that median survival for the entire group was 2 months for those that received antibiotics within 1 month of starting immunotherapy versus 26 months with no prior antibiotic exposure. It is important to note that they observed no difference in survival if the antibiotics were started after immunotherapy had been initiated. That may mean that having the microbiome (the ecosystem of bacteria and yeasts in the gut) intact for the starting dose may be protective even if the microbiome is negatively altered after.

Unfortunately, standard probiotics do not offer any protection and even slowed the recovery of the microbiome after antibiotic therapy. In a 2015 study by Zitvogel published in *Science*, she showed changing the bacteria of the gut (microbiome) could impact the success of immunotherapy in mice. In 2017, further work that she published in *Science* looked at human cases and how the use of antibiotics was linked with lower success and shorter lifespans. This is a very hot topic of study in cancer immunotherapy. It is clear that the bacteria in the gut play an important role in the response to immunotherapy. Some estimate (including myself) that many patients are missing out due to not having the appropriate bacteria, and if this were addressed, the success rates may double. We cannot put a good estimate on this right now, and as therapies improve, it will probably be even more critical. I would estimate that having the correct bacteria in the gut, even without immunotherapy, may be able to prevent cancer, which probably could save the lives of tens, if not over 100 thousand lives a year. That is something to take notice about. Now I need to explain what you can do to enhance your chances of an optimized microbiome.

What are the key bacteria identified to enhance immunotherapy? In a study published in the November 5, 2015 edition of *Science*, Sivan, et al. demonstrated that *Bifidobacterium* were essential for the function of anti-tumoral immunity involving anti-PD-1/PD-L1 immune checkpoint inhibitors. This is very important for the currently popular drugs Opdivo and Keytruda. More than just *Bifidobacterium* in general, it was indicated that the specific species were *Bifidobacterium longum* and *Bifidobacterium breve*. What this means is that Bifidobacterium, especially those containing the *longum* and *breve* species, should be supplemented in any cancer patient's therapy.

How do you do that? *Bifidobacterium* can be purchased over the counter, but it is essential to buy it refrigerated. In any other form, it may not be as potent as more of the bacteria will die. It can also be found in yogurts made with live cultures, fermented foods such as kimchee and sauerkraut (though many of these fermented foods have been pasteurized, so only homemade or artisanal products are likely to contain the living *Bifidobacterium*), some miso, tempeh and umeboshi (a Japanese fermented plum). Whatever form you find it in, always consult with your physician about how to incorporate *Bifidobacterium* into your diet, but do include a refrigerated capsule or powder form a few times a week to ensure you are consuming the correct amount prescribed by your doctor and that it includes significant quantities of *Bifidobacterium longum* and *breve*.

In addition, you need to make sure that these bacteria are fed properly. Certain diets will affect the composition of the gut flora, particularly the standard high fat American diet, which I suggest you avoid. To ensure that the good bacteria are fed properly, make sure to use a daily prebiotic that contains oligofructose or FOS. Studies have shown that increased diversity of the bacteria in the microbiome was another indicator of improved responses to immunotherapy. This was discussed in an article by Gopalakrishnan (*Science* Jan 5, 2018). In general, work published by Dr. Jennifer Wargo from MD Anderson has pointed mostly at a high fiber diet for increasing diversity. The types of fat will also affect the microbiome. Menni, et al. published an article in *Scientific Reports*, September 2017 showing that omega-3 fatty acids are important for microbiome diversity, in addition to a high fiber diet.

There have been several recent studies further investigating gut bacteria (microbiome) and the overall associated treatment success with immunotherapy. Studies published in the November 2017 issue of *Science* by Zitvogel, Routy, et al. demonstrated that the gut bacteria *Akkermansia muciniphila* was the key to turning mice that did not respond to immunotherapy into ones that did. These same bacteria have been an important topic in the past when it comes to obesity, as a higher amount within the gut is found more often in thinner people as compared to ones that are obese. However, this is a separate issue when it comes to cancer. It seems that this bacteria is involved in eating mucus in the gut. Though an increase of Akkermansia muciniphila results in actual increased mucus along the intestinal lining, it seems to increase the interaction of beneficial bacteria with the intestinal wall and at the same time, reduce issues of bacteria permeability of the intestinal wall, known as "leaky gut", which increases inflammation in the body from bacterial substances crossing the bowel wall into the blood stream.

Since this bacterium, Akkermansia muciniphila is so important, how do you make sure that you have enough? Well that is the complicated part. It does not exist currently in probiotics. However, certain pre-biotics that I mentioned containing fructo-oligosaccharides were shown to increase this beneficial bacteria. In an article published by Dr. Kequan Zhou, Wayne State University in *Journal of Functional Foods*, March 2017 titled "Strategies to Promote Abundance of Akkermansia Muciniphila, an Emerging Probiotics in the Gut, Evidence from Dietary Intervention Studies," he outlines diet and supplement changes. Again, a high fat, typical "American" diet is very bad and reduces the numbers of these bacteria. In his article, he cites studies of polyphenols and specifically points to cranberry extract as being able to increase fecal A. muciniphila. Also, very interesting is that Dr. Zhou also references studies of Metformin to increase A. muciniphila, which is commonly incorporated in cancer treatments. The anti-cancer effects of Metformin have mostly been attributed to inhibition of the mTOR pathway and not for glucose control as many would think. It may be that the anti-cancer actions of Metformin are more firmly rooted in the effect on the microbiome. This is becoming a common theme with so many substances that have demonstrated anti-cancer properties. We are now discovering their effects on the microbiome may be their key action.

One other interesting aspect in the article by Dr. Zhou mentions studies supporting Rhubarb extract, which has been reported to have anti-cancer properties, and also shows positive benefits on the microbiome, including increasing A. muciniphila. Rhubarb extract may be another supplement for cancer patients to put on their essentials list.

For many years there has been a group of integrative doctors promoting the use of pancreatic enzymes for the treatment of cancer. Needless to say, this has been met with much controversy. Much of this is related to an embryologist named Dr. John Beard, whose work dates back to the early 1900's. It seems that the work of Dr. Beard was forgotten until the late Dr. Nicholas Gonzalez resurrected it in the 1980's. Though there may be different theories on how pancreatic enzymes may have anti-cancer properties, one very interesting aspect is in article published by Nishiyama, et al., in *Biochemical and Biophysical Research Communications*, October 2017. This article called "Supplementation of Pancreatic Digestive Enzymes Alters the Composition of Intestinal Microbiota in Mice" shows that treatment of mice with a commercially available pancreatic enzyme mixture called Lipacreon, (*EA pharma*, Japan) had a significant increase in Akkermansia muciniphila, 58x greater than controls. I am not implying this may be the only benefit from pancreatic enzyme therapy, but in regards to what we know about the microbiome and the immune response to cancer, this certainly may be an important underlying aspect of its mechanism.

In addition, a study published in the November 27, 2015 edition of *Science* by Vétizou, et al.[5], demonstrated that *Bacteroides* species were important in the function and reduction of side effects in CTLA-4 inhibitors, like the currently approved Yervoy. This information is important because the combination of PD-1/PD-L1 and CTLA-4 is already showing significant enhancement of the anti-cancer immune response over either therapy alone, but side effects can be a problem. This study specifically points to the *Bacteroides* species *B. thetaiotaomicron* and *B. fragilis* as being key to improving the anti-cancer immune response and reducing side effects, specifically associated with colitis. One key aspect to *Bacteroides*, like A. muciniphila, is that these specific bacteria are not included in any normally available probiotics, probably because they do not survive well. One future possibility for enhancing these types of bacteria may turn out to be directly infusing them into the colon through an enema. As of this moment there are not any commercially available forms of enemas containing *Bacteroides* or A. muciniphila, but maybe in the near future there will be.

Along these lines, there is work being done with fecal transplantation. This involves taking stool from one person and transplanting it into another person. The idea is that the donor would be someone that has an excellent microbiome. The best source is someone who had cancer and was treated successfully with immunotherapy. Currently this is not common practice, and the FDA regulations are not clear. Drug companies are rushing around as well to see how they can get into the microbiome game. Thankfully, we have better testing now available. I personally use MicrobiomeDx, to evaluate the microbiome of our patients. Generally my experience has been if the patients make the recommended diet, prebiotic, and supplement changes, they seem to be able to change their microbiome to a more favorable diversity. Certainly it is important not to blow your chance of success with immunotherapy by ignoring a poor microbiome. Treating your gut should be the foundation to any cancer treatment.

Cashew Nuts

Finally, while it may seem nuts, eat your cashews! One of the most intriguing areas of research in the field of probiotics and cancer has been the role that anacardic acid plays in activating immune cells. Anacardic acid is an active component found in cashew nut shell extract and the cashew apples. As far back as 1993, while testing the anti-tumor activity of prostaglandin synthetase inhibitors, Kubo, et al.[6] found that the juice from the cashew tree apple had significant anti-tumoral properties against BT-20 breast carcinoma cells. Cashew apples are commonly found in Brazil, but rarely available in the United States. The active ingredient in this juice that intrigued the researchers is anacardic acid, which is also found in cashew nut oil, and to a lesser degree, in cashews themselves.

Kubo, et al.'s findings have been supported as recently as 2016, when Hollands, et al.[7] were researching multi-drug resistant bacterial strains to address antibiotic resistance. In the process, they found that anacardic acid stimulates the production of reactive oxygen species and neutrophil extracellular traps, which in turn kills harmful bacteria and triggers cell death pathways, boosting innate immune defense.

In a study of the role immune checkpoint inhibitors play in melanoma Frankel, et al.[8] found that positive response to immune checkpoint inhibitors were associated with the presence of specific gut bacteria which induced the maturation of T cells and dendritic cells. In the process of conducting the study, however, they were surprised to discover that those who responded best had high levels of anacardic acid. The researchers concluded that anacardic acid activates immune cells.

While the research on anacardic acid remains limited and in its infancy, I'm persuaded that increasing anacardic acid in the diet through daily consumption of cold-pressed cashew nut oil (or organic cashew butter if the oil can't be found) cannot hurt and has the potential to play a powerful role in enhancing gut flora and immunity. At the very least, adding a once a week serving of cashew nuts may provide a tasty way to boost the immune system and improve gut health. The reason I say once a week is that is what was reported that the patients were taking in the study. I would be cautious not to overdo the cashew nuts, as they are known to be high in lectins, which can damage the lining of the gastrointestinal tract. There certainly could be a consideration to take anacardic acid supplement, which will help avoid the issues of lectins. I am not sure if any exist, but it is a good thought. Another interesting nutrient is Spermidine, which can be found in wheat germ, fermented soy (Natto), soybeans, aged cheese, mushrooms, peas, nuts, apples, pears and broccoli. Studies by Kiechl, et al. (2018) *Am J Clin Nutrition* indicate that Spermidine improves immune surveillance related to cancer.

Despite our growing awareness of the role probiotics play in gut health, at this point we do not have a clear understanding of the precise mechanism that enables bacterial flora to enhance the immune response. One reason we do not yet have a more clear understanding of this mechanism is that other variables affect how they work, including genetics and the distinctive microbiotic diversity that each human gut contains. The most likely possibility is that these bacteria produce specific substances that interact with the immune cells of the intestines. It is this interaction that is key to determining if an anti-cancer immune response will be generated. Pharmaceutical companies are already looking to see if specific bacteria species or genetically modified bacteria can be produced to further enhance the immune response. It is almost certain they will produce such bacteria, but for now, make sure to take the appropriate pre-biotics and other supplements that will give you the best chance for your cancer immunotherapy to work.

In addition to mentioning things that you may want to add to your diet, there are also things that you should consider avoiding. There are numerous chemical, preservatives, artificial sweeteners added to our diet, and often these are hidden. These substances can play havoc with our microbiome. Many people are aware that glyphosate, the primary ingredient in the weed killer known as Roundup, is found as contaminates in food. There have been some studies showing that even at low levels glyphosate affects the microbiome, so avoiding it by eating organic is best. In addition, the artificial sweetener Sucralose, which goes under several brand names, including Splenda, also affects the bacteria in your intestines. Since the name Sucralose is very similar to sugar sucrose, some people may pass it by as an ingredient. After I began searching, I found it in many places that I would have never expected, including vitamins and supplements, so keep your eye out for it and avoid it.

It has seemed in the past couple of decades we have started a war against bacteria, making everything possible anti-microbial. It sounds like we are being protected from bad bacteria out to kill us, but we may be undermining our own health by killing our friendly bacteria as well. The antimicrobial agent Triclosan is found in toothpaste, hand soap, kid's toys and kitchen supplies. However studies are supporting this may be killing your good bacteria as well, leading to a microbiome that may reduce our ability to fight cancer, plus maybe even increasing other conditions such as colitis and inflammatory bowel. In a study published May 2018 by Yang, et al. in *Science Translational Medicine*, they showed that Triclosan altered gut bacteria in mice and treatment with 80 ppm in the diet for 3 weeks reduced the abundance of *Bifidobacterium* by 75%, and you remember how I described earlier in this chapter that *Bifidobacterium* are a key group needed for an anti-cancer immune response. It is best to avoid Triclosan if you can. However, of great concern, as they stated in their article, "Triclosan exposure is practically unavoidable in the United States."

As you can see, basically anything that can function like an antibiotic in the intestines will affect the microbiome. Though things like glyphosate, sucralose and triclosan are not antibiotics per se, they do act like them when ingested.

Controversy of Probiotics

As you have read in this chapter, having the right microbiome not only supports your own natural anti-cancer immunity, but also may be essential to gain success from today's cancer immunotherapy treatments, such as the immune checkpoint inhibitors, Opdivo, Keytruda and Yervoy. One aspect that I would like to emphasize here is that you should not rely on any of these prebiotic and probiotics alone to treat your cancer. Once cancer has developed, it has a good defense network and only in a rare minority of cases would these changes alone make the difference to trigger an anti-cancer immune response by itself. It does happen, but when you hear stories about a patient being cured with diet and/or supplements, it probably means in that patient their immune system was primed and just needed a little push. Though possible, it would be very unlikely that diet and supplements are enough by themselves to result in a cure. They are certainly worth doing, but don't put all your eggs in one basket and delay other treatments.

One key aspect that is coming up in new research is that one of the most important indicators of a microbiome that may promote the most success with immunotherapy is diversity. This means having many types of different bacteria. Because of this, the research is suggesting that overzealous use of probiotics may actually reduce diversity. That being said, we recommend using probiotics just 3-4 times a week, mainly focusing on the additional supplementation of *Bifido breve* and *longum*, just enough to provide some extra, but hopefully not reduce the diversity. If you take too much of specific probiotics, you may reduce your diversity to favor more of the bacteria in the probiotics. Also, some studies suggest that with *Bifidobacterium* it is not necessary to increase the colonization of the bacteria in your intestines because the pass through effect of the bacteria may be just as important. Studies by Wargo show that probiotic supplementation may reduce diversity. She has also shown that microbiome diversity is one of the most important aspects to immunotherapy success. One issue is that there are so many types of probiotics and not much standardization. This makes accurate research difficult. Keep in mind that certain probiotics may be very useful in treating certain autoimmune conditions and colitis, but in immunotherapy we are hoping to generate essentially an autoimmune state against the cancer, so those formulations may not be the best in cancer treatment.

At the SITC 2018, Jobin presented an animal study showing increased colon tumor growth in the mouse model when using the probiotic, VSL#3. This is a probiotic that does very well for inflammatory diseases of the colon, even preventing transition to cancer. However, as this study suggests in mice, once the cancer is there, it may increase growth. So again, I advise caution. The new research has certainly caused me to change my position on probiotic use until we have further data. At least in regards to any general probiotics. However, I think supplementation with *Bifido breve* and *longum* remains important. Based on the research by Wargo, the main goal for any patient should be diversity. This is best achieved by a high fiber diet. In addition, Menni, et al. published Sept 11, 2017 an article in *Scientific Reports* titled "Omega-3 Fatty Acids Correlate with Gut Microbiome Diversity and Production of N-carbamylglutamate in Middle Aged and Elderly Women". Omega-3 is often recommended for cancer patients, and this probably further supports that it may be helpful in increasing diversity of the microbiome. In patients who have done everything they can do for their microbiome and still fail immunotherapy, fecal transplant may be another consideration if their microbiome remains suboptimal. Of course, there are many other aspects beyond the microbiome alone, so I don't want to make you think that it's the only answer. The most important is probably being able to convert a "cold" tumor into a "hot" one.

Again, discuss any of these recommendations with your doctor before trying them on your own. I am listing my basic recommendations later in this book in my "Cancer Immunotherapy Pyramid", though I will not get into specific dosing. Often dosing is not well known and the dosing we use is inferred from studies. Also know that these recommendations often change, so follow my website or blogs to look for any new updates.

Dr. Williams's Microbiome Supplements

1. Prebiotic containing FOS (once daily)
2. Probiotics, one high in *Bifidobacterium*, especially *breve* and *longum* (3-4x a week)
3. Cranberry/Rhubarb Extract
4. Pancreatic Enzymes
5. One serving of Cashews or Cashew-related products containing anacardic acid (once a week)
6. Omega-3

And now that you have your gut under control, it's time to turn to a few more drugs that you'd never expect could help fight cancer. But that's exactly what they do.

CHAPTER 10

Unexpected Off-label Drugs To Boost Your Immunity

THERE HAVE BEEN some remarkable discoveries about how a few different pharmaceutical drugs never intended for cancer treatment turn out to boost immunity in a few different ways and we have found that by including some of these drugs as part of a patient's treatment plan, the chances of fighting cancer improve significantly. Several of the drugs that I've had amazing results incorporating into patient treatment include aspirin, Sitigliptin (a drug for treating diabetes), and believe it or not, Cialis—a drug for erectile dysfunction. In addition, there are several other drugs approved for other purposes than cancer, which may boost the immune response. How do they help fight cancer? Let me explain.

Aspirin

You might not realize it, but early forms of aspirin have been used to treat fevers and pain for the last 2,400 years. Its origins can be traced to the common willow tree, whose barks and leaves have been used medicinally by Native Americans, ancient Egyptians, and ancient Greeks as far back as the 5th century, B.C., when Hippocrates first wrote of it. The bark contains an amazing chemical called salicin, which was chemically isolated in the early 19th century. Unfortunately, the pure chemical also caused serious stomach upset, so it had limited use. But by the late 19th century, while working for Bayer laboratories, German chemist Felix Hoffman created a synthetic form of the chemical from the *spiraea* plant, which also had a long history of traditional medicine use, and was much easier on the stomach. The chemical, acetylsalicylic acid, proved effective for pain relief, inflammation and fevers. Affixing an a- to *spiraea*, and dropping the Latin ending for a simple "n", aspirin was born. Aspirin is now one of the most frequently used medicines in the world and used to treat not only headaches, but also arthritis, heart attacks and yes, even cancer.

Aspirin hasn't changed much in the last century since Hoffman and Bayer Corporation invented it, but what we know about it has evolved. Aspirin is classified as a non-steroidal anti-inflammatory drug (NSAID). NSAIDs are a group of drugs that reduce pain and inflammation, and have even been proven to reduce colorectal cancers.[9] Along with aspirin, Ibuprofen and Naproxen (brand name Aleve) are among the NSAIDs, which act by inhibiting the activity of the enzymes cyclooxygenase-1 (COX-1) and cyclooxygenase-2 (COX-2). Why is that important? It's important because

COX-1 and COX-2 are often elevated in some cancers and they contribute to the synthesis of prostaglandins. One of these prostaglandins, prostaglandin E2 (PGE2), helps tumors to survive, thrive and grow, while simultaneously suppressing the immune system. PGE2 also inhibits the production of interferon and other substances that enhance the anti-cancer T cell response. In other words, by taking aspirin, COX-1 and COX-2 are suppressed which in turn suppresses the production of PGE2, which makes it that much harder for the tumors to survive and spread.

Studies have shown that a combination of immune checkpoint inhibitors and aspirin can reverse the tumor's ability to escape the immune response[10]. This effect did not occur in the absence of aspirin therapy. Despite this important finding, however, the use of aspirin in the treatment of cancer is often underutilized.

There are some doctors who recommend the medication Celebrex, which is classified as an NSAID, but inhibits only COX-2 and not COX-1. But inhibiting COX-2 is important. Hennequart, et al. have noted that COX-2 and its byproduct, PGE2, promote the expression of indoleamine 2, 3-dioxygenase (IDO1) which plays an important role in shielding tumors from immune attack; by inhibiting COX-2, that shield is weakened.[11] IDO1 is responsible for breaking down the amino acid tryptophan, which is needed by immune cells. Essentially it is the food for the immune cells, and IDO is used to starve them. The findings by Hennequart give further insight into the mechanism of how Celebrex may be effective in suppressing tumors. Although inhibiting COX-2 is often effective, however, the early evidence indicates that blocking both COX-1 and COX-2 is important. Consequently, an NSAID such as aspirin, which blocks both COX-1 and COX-2 would theoretically be superior to Celebrex. Although the research remains in early stages, my conclusion is that in many cases aspirin may be a more effective choice than Celebrex. The benefits of Celebrex cannot be ignored; however, for patients with stomach sensitivities to NSAIDs or who otherwise cannot take aspirin, Celebrex remains a good option.

One thing to keep in mind, however, is that dosage is important, as well as how that dosage is administered. The studies with mice that found a reduction in tumor growth after receiving Celebrex were those given dosages of up to five to ten times the standard dose. For this reason, I have found that delivering NSAIDs, such as Celebrex, directly into a tumor may be a better option than taking it orally. One study demonstrated that injecting a hydrogel combined with Celebrex and an anti-PD-1 drug (such as Opdivo or Keytruda) had significant anti-tumor effects[12]. The mouse study showed a 90% reduction in the injected tumor, demonstrating a complete response. It is important to note that the use of the hydrogel was necessary to maintain a higher concentrated, extended release in the tumor microenvironment. This high level of Celebrex seems necessary to have significant benefit and cannot be achieved with oral dosing. But direct injection resulted in a significant decrease in immune suppressive cytokines and inhibited regulatory cells, which in turn gave the immune system a tremendous boost in fighting cancer.

Another study published in the British *Journal of Anaesthesia*, showed that the NSAIDs Ketorolac or Diclofenac when used immediately prior to the start of breast cancer surgery reduced the risk of recurrence or metastasis by 6% in comparison to the non-treated patients[13]. It is hard to get an exact feel how treatment with NSAIDs would impact survival, but if you take a rough estimate based on data from the American Cancer Society indicating that 40,000 American women will die from breast cancer, 6% could mean up to 2,500 lives saved each year in the U.S. alone. Also, I want to stress again, especially for breast cancer patients, don't forget Ketorolac for a biopsy. There are not good studies on this, and in cases where cancer has spread, sometimes surgery could be the culprit. This is due to the increase in growth factors that are released. But how do we know in those cases it was not from the biopsy, which was usually done first? It may cause a release in those growth factors and some studies indicate a drastic rise in circulating tumor cells immediately after a biopsy. So, if Ketorolac helps reduce spread from surgery, it is worthwhile to consider for biopsies as well. Many doctors will state that they don't want to use it because of bleeding risk, but that risk seems exaggerated.

One other study demonstrated that not only is Celebrex effective in suppressing COX-2, it also has the potential to help the immune system attack tumors[14]. Although most of the focus on immunotherapy has been associated with T cells, it may turn out that tumor-associated macrophages (TAMs), which play a key role in inhibiting the anti-cancer immune response, determine whether or not immune checkpoint inhibitors are successful. In a study by Nakanishi, et al., it was shown that by inhibiting COX-2, tumor-protecting TAMs (M2) could be converted into tumor-attacking (M1) TAMs. That means that Celebrex may enhance the anti-cancer immune response.

To date, there have not been comparable studies of the effectiveness of injecting aspirin directly into tumors, perhaps because although aspirin delivered intravenously is fairly common in Europe, the FDA has not approved aspirin for IV use in the U.S. Nonetheless, one study has shown that aspirin delivered intravenously is effective in treating migraine headaches,[15] suggesting that injecting aspirin may be more effective than taking it by mouth for other conditions.

In my practice, I advise my patients to take two full-strength (325mg) aspirin each morning, and again each evening. In some cases I will prescribe two Celebrex (200mg each) along with 650mg of aspirin. When prescribing such high doses of aspirin, however, it's important to monitor the patient for any stomach problems or bleeding. In addition, I am cautious to start the patient on aspirin prior to any procedures due to the increased risk of internal bleeding.

Despite its effectiveness, aspirin is not appropriate for all patients. Side effects can include nausea, vomiting, rashes, and kidney impairment. Aspirin can also worsen asthma, and cause internal bleeding (in the stomach, intestines and brain), and increase the risk of a perforated ulcer. Children and adolescents should not take aspirin at all, because there is a risk of their developing Reyes Syndrome, which affects the brain and liver.

Given these health risks of aspirin, taking high dosages as part of a cancer treatment regime should only be done with the direction and supervision of your physician. Again, do not try this on your own.

As effective as aspirin or Celebrex have proven to be in treating tumors, we still have our work cut out for us when it comes to treating cancer. That is because the microenvironment in which cancer grows is complex and a variety of variables can affect whether a tumor grows or slows. One of the most important of these microenvironmental factors is the acidity of the tumor's environment. If the environment is too acidic (lower pH), the tumor may thrive. But there are a few key steps the physician can take to increase the pH and reduce acidity and thus inhibit the tumor's growth, and in the next chapter, I'll tell you what these steps are and how your physician can help you to control the microenvironments of your own body.

Sitigliptin

When the pharmaceutical company Merck first marketed a phosphate salt under the brand name of Januvia in 2006, they probably never thought it would turn out to have powerful anti-cancer properties. That's because the drug, generically known as Sitigliptin, was an effective treatment for diabetes. Essentially, what it does is inhibits an enzyme called dipeptidyl peptidase 4 (DIPP-4). DPP-4 inhibits gastrointestinal hormones that play a critical role in insulin release; thus, Sitigliptin has been quite effective in controlling diabetes.

DIPP-4 doesn't just contribute to diabetes, however. It also helps tumors to survive and grow. It's so effective in helping tumors grow, in fact, that the tumors themselves appear to increase the production of DIPP-4 as a protective mechanism— think of DIPP-4 as yet another line of defense for tumors. DIPP-4 breaks down and deactivates cytokines, substances that stimulate the immune system, and help immune cells to migrate to areas of inflammation, which includes tumors.

So when treating a patient for cancer, it helps to increase cytokines, and decrease DIPP-4. And now we've found a way to do just that. In a study at the *Institut Pasteur* in France in 2015,[16] researcher Matthew Arnold and his team found that by giving Sitigliptin to mice orally the cytokine CXCL10 increased, which helped attract T cells, NK and dendritic cells to the areas around the tumor, thereby inhibiting the growth of the tumor. More importantly, Sitigliptin inhibited DIPP-4 production and when combined with the immune checkpoint blockers like the CTLA-4 and anti-PD-1 drugs, there was a complete cure in the animal model.

Consequently, when treating patients for cancer, using the combination of anti-CTLA-4 and anti PD-1 medications, I generally prescribe a four-week supply of 25 to 50mg of Sitigliptin taken by mouth starting on the day of ablation or immunotherapy. I have them take the medication for seven days, then go off it for seven days, then go back on it for another seven days, continuing to rotate seven days on and seven days off until the four-week supply is gone.

But that's not all I give my patients. Believe it or not, Viagra, Cialis and Levitra can do more than just save your sex life. These drugs just may save your entire life.

Viagra, Cialis and Levitra

What do Post-It notes and Viagra have in common? They both had strange beginnings, and what was initially considered a failing feature, turned out to be the very feature that made them so successful. When a scientist with 3M set out to make a super-strong adhesive, he failed miserably—the adhesive barely stuck. The story of what happened next varies from secretaries using the adhesive-backed strips of paper to affix easily removable notes to their bosses on documents they typed, to someone using them to mark pages in a book. But whatever the story, the qualities that made the adhesive such a failure were the very qualities that made it such a success—it was an adhesive that didn't stick, at least not for very long. That might not have made it useful for the original intended use, but it made it spectacularly useful for an unintended use.

As for Viagra, the brand name of Sildenfil, it was a drug that was intended to treat hypertension (high blood pressure) and angina (chest pains). It did work for that, but it had a curious side effect—men taking it reported prolonged erections. But what is one man's side effect, is another man's happy evening. Patented in 1996 for treatment of hypertension, by 1998 the FDA approved Sildenfil for erectile dysfunction and soon after two other similar drugs for treating erectile dysfunction came along—Cialis and Levitra.

How can they help treat cancer, you ask, and are they safe for women? Yes, they are safe for women and I'll get to that in a moment, but here's how they work on your immune system and give you a boost in fighting cancer.

Viagra, Cialis and Levitra are all members of a class of PDE-5 drugs. That means that one of their own "side effects" is that they reduce MDSCs (myeloid-derived suppressor cells), which is exactly what you want if you want your immune system to take on those tumors.

MDSCs are similar to the T regulatory cells we discussed in Chapter 2. Remember how they work as screening agents, determining if something was a friend or foe, and were easily tricked by the clever cancer that pretended to be a friend and belonged in the body? Well, like T regulatory cells, MDSCs also interfere with anti-tumor immunity, and they do so by using L-Arginine metabolism to suppress immunity.[17]

Arginine is an amino acid critical to a healthy immune system because it is required to activate T cells. But when cancer is present, tumors and regulatory immune cells produce an enzyme called Arginase 1 which breaks down arginine in the tumor microenvironment.

But one thing that controls this process is the Phosphodiesterase-5 inhibitors, otherwise known as PDE-5. PDE-5 inhibitors reduce the myeloid-derived suppressor cells (MDSCs), and suppress arginase production, which means that tumors have one less ally in their quest to grow and reproduce.

The role MDSCs play in the immune response is a hot topic right now in cancer research, though currently there are no available treatments specifically for controlling them. At present, the best source of PDE-5 and Arginase 1 inhibitors currently available are the popular drugs for erectile dysfunction, Viagra, Cialis and Levitra.

And yes, women can take them safely. They haven't proven to increase arousal as some women (and drug marketers) had hoped, but just as they stimulate blood-flow to the penis, they can stimulate blood-flow to women's genitals, which can increase sensitivity to stimulation. And that's not such a bad side effect when the payoff is increasing stimulation of the immune response for a woman battling cancer.

These drugs, as in any other treatments discussed in this book, need to be taken under the supervision of your physician. Drugs such as Viagra, Cialis and Levitra can cause significant decreases in blood pressure. Patients with low blood pressure may not be able to use them.

Dipyridamole

Dipyridamole is a drug used to treat coronary and peripheral artery disease. It reduces clots and dilates blood vessels. A study published by Rhodes, et al. in *Lancet*, March 23, 1985 demonstrated that melanoma patients given 300mg of Dipyridamole a day had a 5 year survival of 77%, versus an expected survival of 32% in patients not treated with Dipyridamole. One initial thought was that since this drug reduces platelet aggregation, it might decrease the ability of cancer cells to spread in the blood and adhere to other locations, creating metastasis. In a study published by Spano, et al. in *Clinical & Experimental Metastasis,* January 2013, titled "Dipyridamole Prevents Triple-negative Breast-cancer Progression," they demonstrate in the mouse model that Dipyridamole decreased the primary tumor by 67.5% and metastasis formation by 47.5%. In their study, they discovered that Dipyridamole produced a significant decrease in tumor-associated macrophages (TAMs) and myeloid-derived suppressor cells (MDSCs), both which boost the anti-cancer immune response. Dipyridamole also results in a decrease in adenosine, which is a metabolic suppressor of the immune system. As this study shows, basically, there are several mechanisms in which Dipyridamole may help enhance the immune response.

Zoledronic acid

Zoledronic acid is often used to prevent fractures from certain bone metastasis, especially in breast cancer. Studies have indicated that zoledronic acid may reduce the future development of bone metastases in breast cancer. On Dec 10, 2010, Coscia, et al. published a study titled "Zoledronic acid repolarizes tumor-associated macrophages and inhibits mammary carcinogenesis by targeting the mevalonate pathway" in the *Journal of Cellular and Molecular Medicine*. This and studies have shown that zoledronic acid can decrease VEGF and reduce tumor-protecting TAMs, both which may enhance an immune response.

Simvastatin

Simvastatin is an HMG-CoA reductase inhibitor (statin) which inhibits cholesterol synthesis. Several studies, including one by Liu, et al., published in *Sci Rep*, Dec 14, 2015, have shown that Simvastatin can reduce IL-6 production, which is a cytokine that can result in immune suppression. There have been other studies that show this effect may be further enhanced when combined with curcumin.

Rapamycin

Rapamycin is an inhibitor of mTOR which blocks glucose metabolism and cell proliferation. This drug is dose dependent and can result in increased Treg cells, which we do not want. In addition, it can lower proliferation in immune cells, just as well as cancer does. Therefore, although it shows promise as an anti-cancer agent, its use must be closely monitored by a physician.

Metformin

Metformin is a very popular diabetic medication that causes the increase uptake of glucose in muscles and reduces glucose production. It also inhibits mTOR which results in decreased cell proliferation. It enhances T cell killing of cancer, causing tumor shrinkage.

Mepazine/Biperiden

Mepazine is a phenothiazine antipsychotic medication. Biperiden is a medication used to treat Parkinson's disease and is a synthetic acetylcholine antagonist. Both of these drugs inhibit MALT1, which is associated with the CBM signalosome complex. Pilato, et al. published an article in *Nature Research;* Oct 2018 titled "Targeting the CBM Complex Causes Treg Cells to Prime Tumours for Immune Checkpoint Therapy." They demonstrated that using Mepazine to inhibit MALT1 could help convert immunologically cold tumors to hot ones. In the animal model, they showed the combination of Mepazine with PD-1 inhibitors causes the development of an anti-cancer immune response with relapse-free tumor control in a model that does not respond to PD-1 therapy alone. This is important, as the majority of cancers do not respond to PD-1 therapy due to a lack of infiltration of attacking immune cells and a predominance of tumor-protecting regulatory immune cells. They also showed that MALT1 inhibition could actually convert regulatory cells into ones that are more tumor-attacking. The big advantage here is that most strategies are to decrease regulatory cells, generally by killing them. This drug may be able to make good use of those regulatory cells in the tumor environment to convert them into attacking the tumor.

Mifepristone (RU-486)

Mifepristone, also known as RU-486 is an anti-progesterone drug, mainly known as "The French Abortion Pill." Because of the controversy and various abortion laws in different countries, this drug, though promising, would be difficult to obtain, even by prescription of your doctor.

It is known that pregnancy creates an immune suppressing condition, so that the mother's immune system will not attack the fetus. This is related to progesterone and progesterone-induced blocking factor (PIBF). It is known that PIBF may have numerous actions that cause immune suppression against cancer, one being decreasing Natural Killer cell function. It is also known that some cancers produce PIBF as a defense against the anti-cancer immune response. Several case reports have discussed patients who failed traditional chemo and immunotherapies who have seen significant improved survival with mifepristone. This was described in cases of lung and kidney cancers, and even cases of glioblastomas (GBM), a highly malignant type of brain cancer. Technically it would be possible to measure PIBF production, which could help determine if this may be an immune suppressor in specific cancer cases. Right now the studies are lacking, but you can certainly infer that mifepristone could be synergistic with other cancer immunotherapies. Hopefully we will see more studies soon.

Thymosin α1

Thymosin α1 (Tα1) is a peptide that enhances immune function in animals without a thymus and seems to enhance immune function in humans as well. Tα1 used in animal studies reversed some aspects of immune suppression related to chemotherapy. It increases T cell function, and the production of immune stimulatory cytokines, such as IL-2 and IFN-g and NK cell activity. In addition, Tα1 up regulates Toll-like receptor 9. Another important mechanism is that Tα1 increases expression of MHC 1, which can counteract a common mechanism that cancer can use to hide from the immune system.

Tα1 is typically used in the treatment of chronic hepatitis. The described mechanisms above certainly give us a reasonable idea that Tα1 may be useful for enhancing the immune response against cancer, though studies remain limited. Tα1 is typically given as a subcutaneous injection, like insulin, usually twice a week.

Mebedazole/Fenbedazole/Levamisole

I was considering adding a small paragraph on Levamisole, since it is a medication that we had previously used in our patients. However, at the time of writing this book there was a lot of information circulating about a gentleman named Joe Tippens who seemed to have unprecedented success treating his cancer with a dog worming medicine named Fenbedazole along with a vitamin and supplement regimen. Certainly these types of situations occur where isolated patients see unique results in their particular case.

One of my colleagues in Mexico told me about Levamisole 4 years ago, and that it was not uncommon to use parasitic worm medicine in cancer patients there. He reported in 10 years, he had one patient that had a complete response using Levamisole in an advanced colorectal cancer. Once in ten years may not seem much, but for that patient, it was a life changer.

In regards to Levamisole, the data was limited, but I did find a 2007 publication by Chen, et al.; titled "Levamisole Enhances Immune Response by Affecting the Activation and Maturation of Human Monocyte-derived Dendritic Cells." There are also some human studies in the early 2000's that showed some synergy with chemotherapy, though nothing extraordinary. We used it for about two years, but the effect was unclear. Also, though Levamisole may have some immune-stimulating aspects, it can cause immune suppression as well. Pulse or intermittent dosing may help avoid some of this immune suppression, but we just did not have good data, nor did we want to risk counteracting other immunotherapy treatments.

In regards to Fenbendazole, I did not find much data, as well, likely because for an inexpensive drug such as this, it may be difficult to get funding for studies. One interesting article published by Gao, et al., *J Am Assoc Lab AnimSci*, titled "Unexpected Antitumorigenic Effect of Fenbendazole when Combined with Supplementary Vitamins" describes that neither vitamins nor Fenbendazole alone had any effect on tumor growth. In addition, they showed that Fenbendazole alone actually increased tumor growth, which is concerning. However, the combination of Fenbendazole plus vitamins given at a higher than normal level resulted in decreased tumor growth. I have very limited experience with Fenbendazole in patients, but I have seen a few that did seem to have increased growth rate. It sometimes happens where a particular drug may work for some and may worsen others. Certainly dosing may be a problem with these agents, as it seems there is a narrow window for the drug being helpful versus harmful.

Hopefully the increased interest created by Mr. Tippens will lead to further studies and better understanding of these drugs so that more people can be helped. I applaud people like Jane McClelland and Mr. Tippens for helping get information out about off-label drugs that may be helpful for cancer patients. Jane's book *How to Starve Cancer* and her Facebook page on "Off-label" medications are definitely worth following.

Now let's turn to baking soda and acid blockers and see how that can add one more powerful component to the anti-cancer cocktail. That is the focus of Chapter 11.

CHAPTER 11

The Acidic Tumor Microenvironment and Metabolic Immune Checkpoint

I N FOOTBALL THEY say, "Games are won and lost in the trenches." This saying implies that it is some of the lesser-known players in non-glamorous positions that make the difference between winning and losing.

In cancer, the trenches are the tumor microenvironment. Progression of cancer usually boils down to one thing, the inability of the immune system to recognize and eliminate it. For cancer to survive, it must evade the immune system. The metabolism utilized by cancer is one way it can keep the immune system at bay. We have described how cancer can recruit immune-suppressing cells, such as MDSCs, Tregs and TAMs. In addition, tumors can engage receptors on immune cells to head off an immune attack, such as PD-1, CTLA-4, TIM-3 and Lag3.

Cancer is also known to have an energy metabolism that generally differs from most normal cells (though not all) and it is the byproducts of this metabolism that can further suppress the anti-cancer immune response. These byproducts give cancer further benefits from using a metabolic method that would be considered inefficient. One hallmark of this form of metabolism is increased acid secretion from the tumor, leading to an acidic microenvironment.

The antacid properties of baking soda have led many people, including physicians, to recommend sodium bicarbonate for cancer treatment. Tumors utilize glucose in a way that generates a large amount of acid, and then they use this acidic environment to their advantage. That is because acidic environments inhibit the immune system, making it difficult for tumor-attacking cells to survive. The generally preferred metabolism of glucose by cancer (aerobic glycolysis) is known as "The Warburg Effect." The Warburg Effect is named after Nobel laureate Otto Warburg, who in 1924 found that tumors metabolize large amounts of glucose for their energy, and this metabolic process produces copious lactic acid, which significantly inhibits the anti-tumor response. In addition, tumors have more acid pumps to keep the acid outside of their cells (where even to the tumor it is harmful) and increase it in the areas surrounding the cancer. It is equivalent to the tumor spraying an immune system repellant around itself. In studies by Brand, et al. (2016)[18], they found that by genetically engineering tumors to produce less lactic acid, the tumors grew at a slower rate because the immune system was better able to attack the cancer cells. Moreover, the acidic pH of the tumor microenvironment reduces the production of cytokines, specifically Interferon Gamma, or IFN-γ. IFN-γ is a cytokine, a protein necessary for cell communication. IFN-γ is important in cancer treatment because it helps produce cancer-fighting T cells. If the pH of the microenvironment is too acidic, T cell function can be almost completely inhibited.

What this means is that in order to maximize the cancer-fighting properties of the immune system, we need to create a microenvironment with low levels of acidity. And that's where baking soda comes in.

In a study by Pilon-Thomas, et al. (2015)[19], oral administration of sodium bicarbonate in the mouse model significantly enhanced the effect of anti-PD-1 and anti-CTLA-4 immunotherapy. But sodium bicarbonate therapy alone did not have a significant effect on tumor growth. When the researchers combined sodium bicarbonate with immunotherapy the results were particularly promising. This finding is important because many people mistakenly believe that increasing the pH in the microenvironments will help treat cancer, but this study suggest that that technique alone is probably not sufficient. Consequently, for patients receiving immunotherapy, sodium bicarbonate is theoretically beneficial. The question is how much baking soda should a person take to reduce the acidic microenvironment sufficiently to inhibit tumor growth?

The amount Pilon-Thomas, et al. recommended is 800mg per kg of weight each day. At that dosage, a 150-pound patient (which is approximately 68 kg), would need to take 54,400mg, or 54.4 grams, of baking soda. With 4.8 grams of sodium bicarbonate in a teaspoon of baking soda, the recommended dosage would be 3.77 tablespoons, or approximately ¼ of a cup. However, a dosage that high could lead to complications, including metabolic alkalosis, which causes nausea, vomiting, muscle weakness, swelling of the feet and ankles, confusion and even congestive heart failure. For that reason, in my practice I use proton pump inhibitors (PPI) to increase the pH (reduce acidity) of the tumor microenvironment.

PPIs are commonly used to reduce acidity of the stomach and to treat gastritis, gastric ulcers and esophageal erosion from gastric reflux. These drugs can also be used to inhibit the amount of acid that tumors excrete and to increase the pH in the tumor microenvironment. Vishvakarma, et al. (2010)[20] demonstrated that Protonix, the brand name for the PPI pantoprazole, not only affected the pH of the tumor microenvironment, as seen with other PPIs, but it also helped convert tumor-associated macrophages (TAMs) from the tumor-protecting form to the tumor-attacking form. This finding suggests that using pantoprazole may do more than just reduce the acidity in the tumor microenvironment; it may have the added benefit of boosting the immune system's tumor-fighting capabilities.

Another anti-acid medication, Ranitidine, which is a histamine receptor 2 blocker, has also been shown to modify the anti-cancer immune response in mouse models. A study published by Vila-Leahey, et al. in *Oncoimmunology*, March 10, 2016 showed that Ranitidine decreased MDSCs and suppressed tumor growth. In addition, Rogers, et al. published a study in *Frontier Immunology*, August 15, 2018 showing that the anti-cancer immune response from Ranitidine was antibody and B cell dependent. The antibody and B cell response has mostly taken a "back-burner" to T cells, but it still may be very important. Ranitidine may be useful for enhancing this untapped area in cancer immunotherapy.

Since it is the tumor's metabolism of glucose that leads to the production of lactic acid, a main immune inhibitor, there are several potential strategies to enhance the immune response by interfering with glucose metabolism.

One important aspect to understand is there is always a balance in cancer treatment. What do I mean by this? Activated immune cells have similarities to cancer; they need rapid metabolism and grow more cells. So, they also metabolize glucose more by glycolysis, just like cancer. This is what I meant in the beginning of the chapter when I said that cancer metabolizes glucose differently than most normal cells, but not all. There is going to be a balance between starving cancer and the immune cells.

3-Bromopyruvate (3BP)

3-bromopyruvate (3BP) is one of the most powerful agents developed that can block glucose metabolism in cancer. However, the cancer treatment world is filled with controversy, and certainly 3BP is no exception. Its story is pretty well documented on the Internet. In full disclosure, I know the person who discovered 3BP, Dr. Young Ko, very well, I consider her a friend. I think the whole situation is fairly tragic.

To give you a brief history, in the early 2000's Dr. Ko, who was researcher at Johns Hopkins, published an article showing she could cure cancer in rats 100% of the time with direct injection of 3BP into the tumors. The news was huge and people thought a cure for cancer had been discovered. Shortly after, Dr. Ko was fired from Johns Hopkins. The reasons were murky. This resulted in close to a decade long battle in to who had the rights to the drug. This certainly hampered its development by any major pharmaceutical company. The mechanism by which 3BP works is that it can block the metabolism of glucose, which keeps cancer from making energy, resulting in its death. In addition, it seems to be more specific to cancer, without causing much harm to normal cells. Sounds like the answer to cancer, doesn't it?

I have a lot of experience with 3BP, maybe more than anyone else. The reality is that 3BP certainly can be a great tool and possibly a good adjunct to immunotherapy as well, but for most patients, it will not be a cure, at least alone. Cancer still seems to find its way around this, using other substances for metabolism to survive. The delivery is not straightforward either, as 3BP is metabolized rapidly, very little actually makes it to the tumor. Also, I must stress (and warn) that many clinics began offering systemic (IV) 3BP. Most cancer patients would not understand this method is less than satisfactory. We know in general this does not work and may even be harmful. Localized treatment with 3BP, such as injection into the tumor, can enhance the immune response, increasing anti-cancer T cells and natural killer cells. My work with it has been with local injection or intra-arterial infusion, including in combination with immunotherapy. Systemic (intra-venous) treatment with 3BP seems to inhibit the immune response, blocking glycolysis in the immune cells, which causes them to change to oxidative phosphorylation (aerobic metabolism) that favors generation of tumor-protecting regulatory cells. In addition, there seems to be a rebound effect, probably the tumors that survive increase their rate of growth, because they felt like they were being starved. This is not far different than some of the effects seen with chemotherapy. Certainly 3BP may have an important role in cancer treatment, probably boosting the immune response, but again, more so when injected into the tumors, or even intra-arterial infusion, but less likely by a systemic approach such as intravenous (IV) administration.

Another aspect in targeting glucose metabolism is the inhibition of the enzyme Lactate dehydrogenase (LDH-A), which is involved in the conversion of pyruvate (breakdown from glucose) into lactate. It is LDH-A that is a key aspect in helping cancer survive at low oxygen levels, adding energy production from glucose. In addition, the lactate produced is a potent inhibitor of many of the cancer-attacking immune cells, enhancing the tumor-protecting ones. So, inhibition of LDH-A is another important future target. Two agents being studied as LDH-A inhibitors are FX11 and Oxamate.

For more information in relation to tumor metabolism and the immune response, I recommend the article written by Gill, et al.; "Glycolysis Inhibition As a Cancer Treatment and Its Role In An Anti-tumor Immune Response." *Biochimica et Biophysica Acta*: (2016) 1866:87-105.

Reducing the acidity of the tumor microenvironment is just the first step in a complex process of manipulating the microenvironment to be as unfavorable to tumor production and growth as possible, while at the same time maximizing the immune system. Toward this goal, we try to adjust the levels of glucose, oxygen and amino acids. Specifically, we want to reduce the level of available glucose, increase the concentration of oxygen, and increase the amino acid tryptophan in the tumor environment (some other amino acids may actually increase cancer growth).

Tryptophan is metabolized by tumors, and as it breaks down, the immune system is inhibited. Along with this process, an enzyme known as IDO (indoleamine 2,3-dioxygenase) depletes tryptophan levels and inhibits T cell production. This concept led to the development of a tryptophan analog called Indoximod (1-Methyl-D-tryptophan) to inhibit IDO production. By countering the breakdown of tryptophan in the tumor microenvironment with Indoximod, we are able to enhance the anti-cancer immune response. So far studies with IDO inhibitors have not proven to be as successful as originally hoped, but as with many of these agents, it may just be a matter of the right combination, or the right group of patients, or both.

It is important to note that research in the UK by Professor Greg Hannon, of the UK Cancer Institute, Cambridge showed that asparagine, an amino acid that is made by the body, but also found in high amounts in many foods, especially asparagus, increased the growth rate of breast cancer. They suggested a low asparagine diet, or a lowering drug such as L-asparaginase may be more effective because a low asparagine diet is hard to maintain.

As you can see, controlling the complex microenvironments in which cancer thrives is no simple task, but as our scientific understanding of this complex process deepens, we are better able to master the task. By decreasing acidity and increasing essential amino acids, we are better able to starve the tumors and feed the immune system. But without a detailed and holistic understanding of this complex process, standard immune checkpoint inhibitors often fail. Only by balancing the acids, amino acids, glucose and oxygen levels of the tumor microenvironment with precision and expertise can we give the immune system the best chance of defeating cancer. Our scientific knowledge of this process is constantly improving, and it does so at an exponential rate—the more knowledge we gain, the faster our knowledge expands. And that is why the future of immunotherapy is so exciting. We've reached the critical tipping point where a cure for cancer is within our reach. What the future holds for cancer patients is nothing short of remarkable.

If you are interested in learning more on natural and off-label methods to inhibit cancer metabolism, I suggest taking a look at the book by Jane McLelland, *How to Starve Cancer*. Jane is very knowledgeable in metabolic aspects of cancer, and the metabolic checkpoint is certainly a key aspect of cancer immune suppression.

CHAPTER 12

Predicting Immunotherapy Response—Laboratory Testing and Biomarkers

O NE OF THE real challenges in cancer immunotherapy is determining which patients are best suited for immunotherapy and what drugs may be the most effective. I have to admit that our current understanding still leaves much to be desired in this area. One real hope is that with some of the intra-tumoral immunotherapy, understanding and predicting a response may become less important by providing lower risk of side effects, with a higher success rate, lower cost and less investment of time for treatment. Also, some of the intra-tumoral therapies are capable of driving an immune response, even when the markers and other tests are showing a less than favorable chance. One thing to keep in mind is that many of these tests and markers are dynamic and change based on the situation at hand. It may be possible to increase receptors such as PD-L1, often used as predictor to anti-PD-1 therapy. This means that a static test, like PD-L1 staining done on tumor biopsy samples, is probably not the best means for determining a potential response. In addition, the location of where the sample was taken in the tumor, whether in the center or the outer edges, can really change how much expression of PD-L1 that you encounter. Since PD-L1 is a protection mechanism of the tumor against an immune response, you might expect more to be expressed in the peripheral aspect of the tumor, because this is where immune cells would be engaging the tumor, but often biopsies are done in the center. In addition, new studies are showing that tumors may actually excrete PD-L1, which binds and inhibits immune cells even at distant sites from the cancer. In a study published by Guo in *Nature*, August 8, 2018 titled "Exosomal PD-L1 Contributes to Immunosuppression and Is Associated with Anti-PD-1 Response," they showed that tumors facing an immune attack can send out lipid covered PD-L1 to suppress the immune response. As you can see, this is excreted, so it would not be reflected by the tumor biopsy. It is very possible a tumor could excrete PD-L1, but not express much on its own cell surfaces. In these cases, PD-L1 in the blood may be a new indicator of potential immune response to PD-1/PD-L1 inhibitors. At this time, this is not a test that is done to determine if a patient may be a candidate. It is issues such as this where I would suggest great caution in letting some of these tests dictate if a person is to receive a therapy or not. Sadly, some people may be missing out on beneficial therapies due to limited testing available now, which may not always be accurate.

These tests are currently being used in many cases to determine if patients' insurance will provide coverage for immunotherapy. This leaves many patients without the option to give immunotherapy a try, unless of course they pay out of their own pocket. Unfortunately, this may be necessary for a person to receive some of the more cutting-edge treatments. Additionally, most oncologists are sticking to the guidelines and would not be willing to offer it to the patients.

At this time, the typical evaluation for a potential immune response includes Microsatellite instability (MSI)/ Mismatch repair and PD-L1 receptor expression on the tumor. Microsatellite instability (MSI) assesses mutations in DNA that occur from DNA mismatch repair. Sometimes when the DNA is being copied there are mistakes that occur and typically those are recognized by the body and fixed. Just like mistakes in writing, you can have misspelled words, which results from the incorrect letter, or you can have an entire misplaced word. When the cell cannot fix these DNA errors, you get an accumulation of many of them over time. The theory is that the more errors, the greater difference these cells would have from normal cells, hence they would be easier for the immune system to recognize. In colorectal cancers, tumors with high MSI (MSI-H) have a better prognosis, probably related to the immune system's ability to detect them easier. However, keep in mind this is not always the case. Renal cell cancers, for example, often have few mutations, yet still respond fairly well to immunotherapy.

In many cases of cancer, the immune system may still naturally try to fight it and be losing, but if it is fighting, the cancer generally cannot grow as rapidly, which results in a better prognosis. Also in these cases, it is easier to stimulate these into an effective immune response if the immune system is already trying to fight on its own.

Programmed death-ligand 1 (PD-L1) is a membrane bound protein that can suppress an immune response and protects against autoimmunity. This binds to the PD-1 receptor and this interaction is the main target with some of the most popular immunotherapy drugs, such as Opdivo and Keytruda. As mentioned, testing of the tumor sample to evaluate expression of PD-L1 is used to determine potential success and often insurance coverage for treatment with this class of drugs. I think many of the hardcore researchers agree that this is not the most accurate evaluation, as patients whose tumor does not express PD-L1 may also respond, though typically with much less success. In addition, there are many aspects that we do not understand related to these receptors.

There is now a good indication that the timing of when these drugs are administered is important. Basically, you need to increase the initial immune response, the immune system's desire to want to attack the tumor first, then, in certain cases, follow up with PD-1/PDL-1 drugs to boost the response. If the timing is off, the immune response may actually be hindered. It is like starting a car. There is a sequence of events that must happen with fuel, compression, and spark plug ignition. If these happen out of sync, the engine will not start. This is still an area that needs more understanding, but again, intra-tumoral immunotherapy may help solve some of these issues, as previously mentioned with agents like TLR agonist. The TLR agonist seem to be important for getting the car cranked, while the other immunotherapy agents can remove the brake and step on the gas.

Another test that seems to be helpful and certainly will become more widely used is Immunoscore, which was developed by Dr. Jerome Galon in Paris, France. The basic concept of this test is to evaluate the tumor specimen and the associated evidence of an immune response. Essentially, if there is evidence of more intense immune response, a so-called "inflamed tumor," then the prognosis is better. This would be an Immunoscore "4". An "immune desert", meaning an absence of immune cells within the tumor resulting in an Immunoscore "0" has a poorer prognosis. This is essentially a new staging system, which does not depend on tumor size like the old standard system. Also, this test looks at both the center and outer edges of a tumor which, as I mentioned before, is important because immune expression is often different depending on the part of the tumor sampled.

The principle behind Immunoscore is very much the way I feel, as well: staging is based more on how your immune system responds and less on size, location, and the number of tumors. I think a new staging system should be developed taking into account these immune aspects and also the overall tumor volume. In my experience the more tumor volume, the harder the cancer is to treat. We know that cancer produces substances to enhance its growth and suppress the immune system, so the more cancer, the potentially more powerful that effect may be. However, you could have an early stage cancer patient that has more tumor volume than a Stage IV patient. In traditional treatments, the earlier stage patient would have the better prognosis, but with immunotherapy, you could argue that the one with less tumor volume may have the better prognosis. Certainly a patient with less tumor volume and an inflamed tumor microenvironment should have a better prognosis than one with earlier stage disease that is an immune desert. We do believe that we can change a lot of these cases of an immune desert into a favorable inflammatory response within the tumor by the direct injection of immunotherapy agents such as TLR and STING agonist, thus leveling the playing field.

CHAPTER 13

Natural Substances and Supplements to Enhance the Cancer Immune Response

ANY CANCER PATIENTS load up on numerous supplements to help treat their cancer. I certainly agree that many of these may be helpful. I have already discussed several within the other chapters of this book.

There are an endless number of supplements, many with unknown benefits. In this chapter, I would like to discuss some of the more popular ones. I do not always recommend these to my patients, though that does not mean they may be without benefit. I hope to give an objective summary, so that each patient can make their own decision if these are things they may want to add to their treatment protocol.

Cannabis Products

Certainly you cannot delve too far into alternative and natural treatments for cancer without running into people saying that marijuana cures cancer. I have many patients who have tried cannabis products, but I have not personally run into any that were cured from using them. I wanted to know where these people who have been cured are. I attended some meetings with people discussing all the benefits of cannabis. The stories they described sounded promising, at least in the way they tell them to the lay public. But I did not see the real evidence. Many of the cancers they were citing great benefits for are ones that people can generally live with for many years, if not a decade or more. So, stating that a person was still alive after one year of cannabis use was not the results I was looking for.

In regards to the immune response, research has shown that there are receptors in the immune system for compounds found in cannabis called cannabinoids. There are two receptors, CB1 and CB2. CB2 is found on immune cells. In an article published by Rieder, et al. May 20, 2009 in the journal of *Immunobiology*, called "Cannabinoid-induced Apoptosis in Immune Cells As a Pathway to Immunosuppression," they describe that cannabis inhibits the immune system and increases regulatory cells. These are not good things when it comes to cancer. So, how can there be all this information out on the internet that cannabis cures cancer, or at least helps? Certainly it seems helpful with symptoms of cancer, but that does not mean it makes cancer better.

In my research I found that there was a general overall lack of good studies on this topic. At the European Society of

Medical Oncology, September 2017; Taha, et al. presented a poster titled "The effect of cannabis use on tumor response to Nivolumab in patients with advanced malignancies." In their study there were some concerning results related to cannabis use and cancer, showing patient using cannabis with the immunotherapy Nivolumab had a greater than 50% reduction of their response rate (37.5% versus 15.9%).

On the positive side, there have been animal studies with CBD and a human study with THC directly injected into tumors that have had some promising results. Also, cannabis is a complex mixture, containing numerous compounds. It is very possible that specific isolated extracts may have benefits. We still have a lot to learn in regards to cannabis products and the treatment of cancer. Our group plans to conduct further studies looking at the immune response from intra-tumoral injection of cannabis extracts. However, it does seem clear that cannabis products can help with certain cancer-related symptoms, but this is more for palliation and not for actual treatment of the cancer.

Silibinin (Legasil)

Silibinin, which is derived from milk thistle, is used as a liver protector and is sold as Legasil. A study published by Priego, et al. demonstrated that with 18 patients with lung cancer and brain metastases who were given oral Legasil, the response rate in the brain was 75% with 20% demonstrating a complete response. The effect was more impressive in the brain than the body.

Silibinin is an inhibitor of STAT3, which inhibits the immune response by increasing MDSCs and Tregs. STAT3 also promotes the secretion of TGF-B, which as we have discussed is a potent suppressor of the anti-cancer immune response.

6-Gingerol

6-Gingerol is the bioactive ingredient in raw ginger that inhibits arginase and helps convert M2 (tumor-protecting) macrophages into a M1 (tumor-attacking) phenotype. This is an important area of immune resistance and immune checkpoint failure. Also, Lo Russo, et al. showed that macrophages might be an important mechanism that resulted in hyperprogression (rapid cancer growth) with the treatment of PD-1/PD-L1 inhibitors. Hyperprogression is a major concern with this type of immune checkpoint therapy as it results in reduced survival that is actually caused by the therapy when patients are treated with drugs such as Keytruda and Opdivo.

Berberine

Berberine is a plant-derived extract that has been shown to lower blood sugar. Studies suggest in cancer that berberine may inhibit cell proliferation and promote apoptosis. There are other studies, however, that suggest berberine may have immune suppressing effects, which does create concern in cancer treatment. But other studies have contradicted this finding, so berberine's role as a potential anti-cancer agent remains unclear.

Berberine also seems to affect the microbiome, but it is unclear if the effect is beneficial in cancer. Karimi, et al. published a study in *J Acupunct Meridian Stud,* April 2017 that showed in the mouse model that berberine caused a decrease in Treg cells in the spleen and also reduced IL-10, an immune suppressing cytokine. Kim, et al. published a study in *Cell Physiol Biochem*, Jan 31, 2018 that demonstrated that berberine suppressed breast cancer cell motility by decreasing TGF-B, a major immune suppressor.

Selenium

As I had mentioned earlier in this book, I saw a poster presentation at the 2017 SITC by Lennicke, et al. that described how supplementing with selenium could help patients who begin failing PD-1 inhibitors to respond again. There is much in the literature describing the anti-cancer and cancer prevention properties of selenium. However, as I did further research, I discovered that there are a few things to consider. The main supplemental forms of selenium is selenomethionine (SeMet) and, occasionally, selenium-methyl L-selenocysteine. When I reviewed the literature, the more significant effects are seen with methylseleninic acid (MSA). However, I have been unable to locate this in supplement form. Yan, et al. published a study titled "Dietary supplementation with methylseleninic acid, but not selenomethionine, reduces spontaneous metastasis of Lewis lung carcinoma in mice." It does seem there may be some conversion inside the body from SeMet to MSA, but the studies I read still show that the results are inferior. So, for the time being, it seems selenomethionine may be the best option, until maybe MSA becomes available.

Lennicke, et al., published another study in *Oncoimmunology*, Dec 2016 "Modulation of MHC class I surface expression in B16F10 melanoma cells by methylseleninic acid (MSA)." They describe that MSA may increase MHC I expression in tumor cells, which blocks a method that cancer can use to escape the immune response. In addition, MSA seems to have other immune-stimulating effects that decrease regulatory cells and many immune inhibitor substances, like VEGF and PDGF.

Curcumin

Curcumin is a plant-based compound that is a primary active ingredient in the spice turmeric. It has often been used as a supplement in cancer treatments. Bhattacharyya, et al. published in *J BiolChem,* June 2007 their findings that curcumin can protect tumor mediated T cell destruction. In addition to the direct effect on tumor growth, curcumin seems to increase tumor suppressor gene p53 and may enhance the anti-cancer immune response by decreasing TGF-B.

EGCG (Epigallocatechingallate)

EGCG is a polyphenol generally extracted from green tea. This is a supplement that is often used in cancer treatment. I would like to add a warning that there have been reports of liver damage at high doses. Therefore, EGCG should be used with caution. As with anything else discussed in this book, its use should be addressed with your doctor before taking it or engaging in any of these other therapies.

Ogawa, et al. published a study in *OncolLett*, Sept 2012 demonstrating that EGCG may have immune enhancing effects by inhibiting IDO, an enzyme we discussed previously that breaks down tryptophan, which is necessary for immune cell function. Studies have also suggested that the combination of EGCG and curcumin may decrease TGF-B. In addition, several studies have shown that EGCG can inhibit cancer stem cells.

Sulforaphane

Sulforaphane is obtained from cruciferous vegetables, such as broccoli. It is necessary to have enzymatic production of sulforaphane, which is generated when myrosinase converts glucoraphanin into sulforaphane. So, when you are looking for this as a supplement, you will want the activated form. Castro, et al. published a study in *Cancer Prev Res*, March 2019 that reported sulforaphane suppressed breast cancer stem cells. In regards to sulforaphane there may be some contradicting aspects when it comes to the immune response. Some studies suggest it inhibits TGF-B, which can reduce immune suppression in advanced cancers. A study by Johler, et al., *Cancer Immunol Immunother*, Dec 2016 showed that sulforaphane inhibits macrophage migration inhibitory factor (MIF) that can help cancer escape the immune system. Also, inhibiting MIF with sulforaphane can result in a decrease in MDSCs, which should further help the anti-cancer immune response. However, the authors, Liang, et al. published a study in *AdvBiolRegul*, Jan 2019 discussing how sulforaphane may be a "doubled-edged sword" when it comes to cancer immunotherapy. They state that sulforaphane acts pro-oxidatively in human T cells, which can inhibit their activation and tumor killing functions. Clearly, it is hard to say if it is best to take the good with the bad in regards to sulforaphane. In general, I feel the benefits may outweigh the negatives, but we certainly need more studies.

Polydatin

Polydatin is the precursor of resveratrol. New studies, like the one published by Mele, et al., *Cell Death Dis*, May 2018, discuss how polydatin inhibits G6PD, a major glucose metabolism pathway. They showed that polydatin suppressed cancer proliferation and metastasis. Though there is not a lot of direct links as to how this can affect the immune response, I did think it was at least worth mentioning. Remember that glucose metabolism results in significant lactic acid production, creating a metabolic immune checkpoint. Also, there is evidence that Polydatin may decrease the Wnt/beta-catenin pathway, which in theory could result in increased immune cell infiltration in the tumor microenvironment. Clearly more studies are needed, but the theoretical aspects of Polydatin suggest that it may have effective anti-cancer properties and could result in further immune enhancement.

Beta Glucans

Beta glucans, also known as B-glucans, are polysaccharides that come from the cell walls of oats, barley, mushrooms, yeast, bacteria, and fungi. They bind to immune receptors and can attract immune cells into the tumor environment. Depending on where they are derived, B-glucans can have different effects. It is still unclear which source of B-glucans is superior, if any. Theoretically the oat/barley-based B-glucans may have an advantage, but that still is not fully proven. No matter the source, all types of B-glucans seem to have immune enhancing properties. They are able to decrease regulatory cells and increase immune-stimulating cytokines, which can help "turn up the heat" in the tumor microenvironment. Since a cold tumor microenvironment is a major reason for immunotherapy failure, B-glucans have the potential to boost the response of immunotherapy.

As I had mentioned before, the potential list of natural substances that may be immune-stimulating is exhaustive. I selected some of the ones that I thought have the most evidence and potential, without being too overwhelming. A patient can only take so many supplements and medications.

Now that you know about a few immune enhancing supplements, we have to discuss some of the darker side of immunotherapy, adverse reactions. Thankfully we can use intra-tumoral injection to minimize these side effects, while maximizing success and reducing cost.

CHAPTER 14

Immune Related Adverse Events and Side Effects of Cancer Immunotherapy

EVEN THOUGH ONE major goal in cancer treatment is to get away from the terrible side effects of chemotherapy and radiation, immunotherapy is not perfect. I think in general the side effects of immunotherapy are probably better tolerated and have a higher patient satisfaction as compared to chemotherapy. In addition, the overall success rate (which seems to be rapidly increasing with new drug developments) makes some of the side effects of immunotherapy more palatable. Even so, there are a few important issues concerning side effects associated with immunotherapy. One, doctors may not be quick to recognize some of the symptoms, especially since most will occur while the patient is home, so it is important for the patient to be aware so that they can alert their doctor. Two, most of the serious side effects of today's typical immunotherapy are autoimmune related and usually respond to steroids. Three, new drugs and combinations may result in side effects that are more severe, even fatal, and may have a different mechanism than autoimmune issues, which means they may require different treatments than steroids.

Autoimmune Side Effects

We have discussed that with the common immunotherapy drugs used today, mostly anti-PD-1/PD-L1 or anti-CTLA-4, block receptors that prevent your immune system from attacking your own body, it is certainly understood that this can increase autoimmune conditions. In general, you could expect to see any type of autoimmune conditions that may occur in normal disease processes, such as rheumatoid arthritis, Hashimoto's thyroiditis, and colitis. However, with cancer immunotherapy it is possible to see autoimmune issues almost anywhere in the body, and certainly some that would be very strange or extremely rare to occur naturally.

There is a long list of possible autoimmune conditions, but certainly ones to consider are: pneumonitis (lung), hepatitis (liver), thyroiditis (thyroid), colitis (colon), diabetes (pancreas), hypophysitis (pituitary gland), rash (skin). Though I will not go into the detailed treatment of these issues, in many cases, corticosteroid treatment may be necessary. We usually warn our patients that any changes in breathing or shortness of breath could be from pneumonitis, an autoimmune inflammation in the lung. This needs to be evaluated immediately, and my suggestion is with a CT scan of the chest. I would like to mention here that a chest X-ray alone is not very sensitive for picking up this condition. Though it may be the first step, ultimately a CT scan probably will be needed.

It is important to note that the appearance of autoimmune pneumonitis can resemble pneumonia in some cases, but the treatment is clearly different. Every effort needs to be made to distinguish these apart from each other. In general pneumonia (lung infection) will have an elevated white blood count and fever, whereas pneumonitis typically would not. Sometimes the distinction is not so clear.

In regards to thyroid issues, most commonly the autoimmune issue results in a low thyroid hormone, hypothyroid. In some cases this may start as a high or hyperthyroid condition, because the gland is being destroyed by the immune system, which causes a rapid sudden release of thyroid hormone, later followed by a decrease in thyroid hormone production. The increase in thyroid hormone may cause symptoms such as anxiety and a rapid heart rate, which may need to be treated with medicines to control these symptoms, such as a Beta blocker. In other cases the autoimmune antibodies can actually stimulate the thyroid, causing an increased production of thyroid hormone, also known as Grave's disease. This is where the increased thyroid hormone production can persist, unlike the first condition I described of thyroiditis, where hormone levels may first come up, but later become low. In either case, it may be necessary to have an endocrinologist evaluate and treat these situations.

In regards to autoimmune hepatitis, it is important to periodically monitor liver enzymes. Mild increases can just be monitored, but more significant increases will need to be treated with steroids or, in rare cases, other immune suppressing drugs.

There are many different recommendations on how to treat these related autoimmune conditions. I would refer someone to either the prescribing information provided by the drug manufacturer or to consult with their doctor. There are also helpful treatment guidelines on the website www.uptodate.com, which is an evidence-based medicine website used by many physicians. The book *SITC's Guide to Managing Immunotherapy Toxicity* by Ernstoff, et al., published in 2019, is an excellent reference book and a must for the library of any doctor involved in the use of cancer immunotherapy.

Typical Side Effects or Autoimmune Related Events with Immune Checkpoint Therapy

The following reactions are among the most common side effects or autoimmune related events experienced by patients who undergo immune checkpoint therapy:

Fatigue

Skin rash, itching, vitiligo, dry mouth

Diarrhea/colitis

Liver toxicity/hepatitis

Pneumonitis (inflammation of the lung)

Thyroiditis (inflammation of the thyroid)

Hypophysitis (inflammation of the pituitary)

Adrenal Insufficiency

Diabetes

In addition to these reactions, some of the more rare side effects below may become more common in the future with new drugs or combinations. These may include neurological issues and cardiac toxicity. These thankfully seem rare, but when they do occur, they can be very severe. We often do a cardiac evaluation on patients prior to treatment, with monitoring of cardiac enzymes via periodic lab tests after they start treatment.

Again, these are some of the more common issues, but not a complete list. If you are being treated with immunotherapy, do not hesitate to discuss any concerns with your doctor.

Skin rash/itching

Skin rashes and itching may not seem like a major problem, but it can be extremely distressing and annoying for patients. Commonly, if this is in a small localized area, steroid creams can be fairly effective. Using antihistamines can also be helpful. However, the associated itching, especially over a larger area of the body can really be a problem when it does not respond to these conservative treatments. I want to share something that we have had success with, most typically in patients on systemic PD-1/PD-L1 inhibitors. A publication by Ito, et al., in *Lung Cancer,* July 2017 titled "Aprepitant for Refractory Nivolumab-induced Pruritus" describes how aprepitant (Emend), an oral neurokinin-1 receptor antagonist was useful in a case report. We have also used this with fairly good success as well. This medicine is normally used for the prevention of chemotherapy-induced nausea and vomiting. The medication can be fairly expensive if not covered by insurance. Generally it only needs to be used for 3-5 days to have effect. So if you are having issues with itching that are not responding to other treatments, it may be wise to suggest this to your doctor. I would recommend that you show them the above article, which you can find the summary of on the Internet.

Tumor Lysis Syndrome

Though relatively rare, tumor lysis syndrome (TLS) should be considered and monitored for in immunotherapy cases, especially with new immunotherapy combinations in a patient with a heavy tumor burden. TLS can occur when there is a rapid destruction of cancer. It may seem like a good problem to have, but it can become very serious. The rapid destruction causes a release of materials within the cancer into the blood which, if severe and not treated properly, can become fatal. The dead tumor causes an increase in electrolytes, potassium and phosphate, with low calcium, increased uric acid and blood urea nitrogen (BUN). These breakdown products can ultimately lead to kidney failure. Due to these electrolyte issues, this can be monitored by lab analysis.

The treatment of tumor lysis syndrome is well described, and one of the most important aspects is IV hydration. I will add that oncologists are often very surprised that this can occur with immunotherapy. I have seen it in patients and had oncologists delay treatment because they did not feel it was possible. My suggestion, is to make sure to get follow up labs and if the labs suggest tumor lysis, it is best to treat it as such, as soon as possible.

Cytokine Release Syndrome

Cytokine release syndrome (CRS) is one of the most problematic issues in cancer immunotherapy. Originally extremely rare, the incidence of CRS is rapidly increasing, especially with the development of new agents and combination immunotherapy. CRS has given great problems to patients treated with CAR-T, which has been successful in blood born cancers, but carried huge risk. We also began seeing it in more patients, with bulky disease when using combination immunotherapy directly injected into the tumor. Basically, it is a condition caused when the immune cells produce a large amount of immune-stimulating substances called cytokines in response to mounting an immune attack, in this case, against cancer. It seems the larger amount of cancer burden the patient has, the higher the risk there is for CRS. The immune system is used to attacking things that relatively small, such as a viral or bacterial infection that does not have much mass, but cancer tumors can be larger than one of your organs. When the body attacks something so massive it is not without potential consequences.

Symptoms of CRS typically include fatigue, fever, loss of appetite, vomiting, low blood pressure, seizure, headache, and confusion. This is very similar to the symptoms associated with severe infections and sepsis. Fatigue, fever and loss of appetite can be common in immunotherapy, as well, but CRS progresses to these other symptoms, often starting with low blood pressure. For me, this was the major drawback of immunotherapy. I feel it is one reason that it is best to treat patients as early as possible, before their disease becomes too bulky, since increased tumor burden is a risk factor. Other thoughts are to use chemotherapy, radiation, or ablation to reduce tumor volume first, though often this is not possible. However, thankfully, recently some major breakthroughs have been made. They may not eliminate the problem, but hopefully they will make it manageable in most cases.

In a study published in *Nature Medicine*, May 2018 by Norelli, et al. they showed that cells of the immune system called monocytes produce Interleukin 1(IL-1) and Interleukin 6(IL-6) causing CRS in a specific mouse model. Importantly, the study showed that IL-1 seems to be the source of associated neurotoxicity in CRS. This type of toxicity is normally the most dangerous and fatal aspect.

Besides supportive care, the typical treatments for CRS are steroids, histamine blockers, and potentially the IL-6 blocking agent Tocilizumab. However, this last treatment has not been as successful as hoped, especially in a case where neurological symptoms have developed. Norelli, et al. showed that IL-1 seemed to start this whole cascade and was responsible for the neurological toxicity. This led them to show that the IL-1 blocking drug Anakinra did have success in preventing the neurological related toxicity. This was in the animal model, but it is important enough that we should consider using this therapy in patients right away. Thankfully, Anakinra is already FDA-approved for treatment of rheumatoid arthritis, so it can be used off-label in the U.S.

TNF inhibitors

In a study published in *Nature*, May 2, 2019, Perez-Ruiz, et al., described how the prophylactic use of TNF blockers increased the effectiveness of the combination of CTLA-4 and PD-1 immunotherapy, while at the same time reducing autoimmune colitis and hepatitis. Keep in mind, this is in a mouse model, but is still promising. In this study they used the TNF inhibitor etanercept (Enbrel). They showed that not only were adverse autoimmune effects reduced, but also there was increased T cell infiltration in the tumor that resulted in increased complete tumor rejection. Overall this sounds like a "win-win" situation. Though clearly we need further studies, since etanercept is FDA-approved it could easily be adopted as an off-label treatment.

Hyperprogression

Hyperprogression is an actual increase in the cancer growth rate caused from the treatment with immune checkpoint inhibitors (PD-1/PD-L1) such as Opdivo and Keytruda. Reports indicate this may occur in 4-29% of patients treated in multiple cancer types. It is not as clearly defined and can be confused with pseudoprogression, where patients have an initial increase in tumor size first and ultimately a decrease. The degree of tumor increase with hyperprogression is greater than that seen with pseudoprogression, with often a doubling in tumor size and the development of new tumor locations as compared to the pre-treatment and first post-treatment scans. It is important to note that hyperprogression will shorten the patient's lifespan, meaning it will make them worse than if they were not treated at all. Frankly, that is a little scary.

Studies have indicated an association with MDM2 gene amplification and EGFR aberrations. However, these are still not clear. More promising, in a recent study published in *Clinical Cancer Research* by Lo Russo, et al., Sept 11, 2018, they implicated tumor-associated macrophages (TAMs) as potentially being a major culprit. Basically they describe that part of the PD-1/PD-L1 antibody (drugs such as Opdivo/ Keytruda to block these receptors) binds to a part of the tumor-associated macrophages (TAMs) and may actually activate them to become more tumor-protecting. When this part of the antibody (drug) was removed, the enhanced growth rate of cancer was not seen. In the mouse model they also found that using clodronate, a first generation bisphosphonate used for the treatment of osteoporosis (approved in many countries, but not the U.S.), was able to reduce the macrophages and hyperprogression.

As I have mentioned, tumor-associated macrophages may be an important area of immunotherapy resistance. This will be an area that needs to be addressed with combination therapy. Several drugs are in development for this, with one of the most promising being CSF-1R inhibitors. Also, an Anti-MARCO antibody was able to convert the tumor-protecting macrophages into the tumor-attacking type.

As you learned earlier in Chapter 13, 6-Gingerol is a natural substance that can inhibit TAMs, though probably not to the level of these experimental drugs, but at least it is easily available. Clodronate may be an option as well, at least in countries where it is approved. Studies have shown that zoledronic acid (Zometa) has similar effects and is approved in the U.S. The extract from milk thistle, Silibin may also have a role in inhibiting cancer protecting tumor-associated macrophages (TAMs). Also don't forget mangostin, a human STING agonist mentioned earlier, because it not only activates STING, but also converts TAMs from the M2 to M1 type (tumor-protecting to tumor-attacking). However, keep in mind that this would need to be injected into a tumor directly.

In summary, even though the goal of immunotherapy is to have a successful cancer treatment with less side effects of traditional chemotherapy and radiation, there remain many potential serious side effects that can be caused by immunotherapies, as well. These must be monitored and in certain cases may require treatment. It is important for the patient to be aware of these potential issues and notify their doctor immediately if concerning symptoms develop.

CHAPTER 15

Dr. Williams's Cancer Immunotherapy Pyramid and Plan to Maximize Success

I MUST STRESS THAT anything discussed in this chapter or elsewhere in this book should be discussed with your doctor before making changes on your own. It is important to know that what I've shared are general guidelines and they may not be suitable for all patients. Also keep in mind that our knowledge in cancer immunotherapy is growing at an incredible pace, so many new developments may occur. I will try my best to provide updates about new developments on our social media pages. In addition, the list of potential off-label medications and natural substances is exhaustive. It would be impossible for a cancer patient to take everything that has been shown to have anti-cancer properties. Many of these may have theoretical benefit based on laboratory studies, but it is still unknown if that will translate into anything worthwhile in actual patients. Some of these medications are popularized by stories of other patients' success, but keep in mind that each person is unique, so it may not transfer well patient to patient. These off-label medications and natural substances are also used in combinations that are not specifically studied, so the interactions and interference of responses generally are not known. In immunotherapy for cancer, we have to worry that certain medications might gain a patient short-term success at the expense of a long-term cure.

Below are suggestions for potential off-label medications and natural substances to enhance the anti-cancer immune response. The pyramid gives potential agents in different categories to enhance the immune response. This does not mean a person could or should take everything listed. Medications like Cialis and Propranolol lower blood pressure, and some patients cannot take either one, while many would not tolerate both together. **I cannot stress enough that unsupervised use of the listed medications and supplements can be dangerous, so always consult with your doctor before using.**

Again, there are a limitless number of agents that could be on this list, but those that follow are ones that I feel have good scientific data.

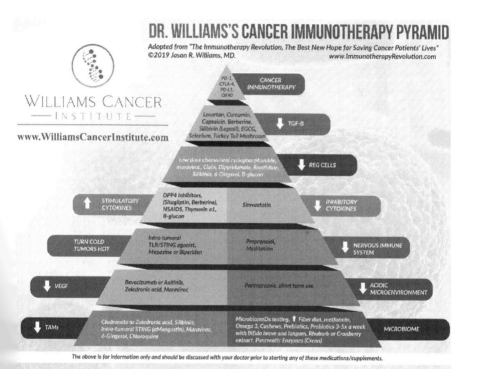

DR. WILLIAMS'S CANCER IMMUNOTHERAPY PYRAMID

Adopted from "The Immunotherapy Revolution, The Best New Hope for Saving Cancer Patients' Lives"
©2019 Jason R. Williams, MD.   www.ImmunotherapyRevolution.com

WILLIAMS CANCER
—— INSTITUTE ——
www.WilliamsCancerInstitute.com

PD-1, CTLA-4, PD-L1, OX40	CANCER IMMUNOTHERAPY
Losartan, Curcumin, Capsaicin, Berberine, Silibinin (Legasil), EGCG, Selenium, Turkey Tail Mushroom	⬇ TGF-B
Low dose chemo/oral cyclophosphamide, maraviroc, Cialis, Dipyridamole, Ranitidine, Silibinin, 6-Gingerol, B-glucan	⬇ REG CELLS

⬆ STIMULATORY CYTOKINES | DPP4 Inhibitors, (Sitagliptin, Berberine), NSAIDS, Thymosin a1, B-glucan | Simvastatin | ⬇ INHIBITORY CYTOKINES

TURN COLD TUMORS HOT | Intra-tumoral TLR/STING agonist, Mepazine or Biperiden | Propranolol, Meditation | ⬇ NERVOUS IMMUNE SYSTEM

⬇ VEGF | Bevacizumab or Axitinib, Zoledronic acid, Maraviroc | Pantoprazole, short term use | ⬇ ACIDIC MICROENVIRONMENT

⬇ TAMs | Clodronate or Zoledronic acid, Silibinin, Intra-tumoral STING agonist(aMangostin), Maraviroc, 6-Gingerol, Chloroquine | MicrobiomeDx testing, ⬆ Fiber diet, metformin, Omega 3, Cashews, Prebiotics, Probiotics 3-5x a week with Bifido breve and longum, Rhubarb or Cranberry extract, Pancreatic Enzymes (Creon) | MICROBIOME

The above is for information only and should be discussed with your doctor prior to starting any of these medications/supplements.

Conclusion

WHEN I SET out to join the legions of men and women who have been working for decades toward a cure for cancer, I knew the ride would be a long one. But I was unprepared for how rapidly advances in our scientific knowledge would speed my journey and bring me to where we are today, where a cure for cancer seems imminent.

But the task remains a challenging one. Not only are the types of cancer complex and diverse, but so, too, will be their treatments. And even more diverse are the patients we treat.

One thing I have learned to appreciate in my practice is that there are numerous factors that can affect a patient's immune response, from their own unique physiology, to their mental state and the social support that they have to help them through their treatment and recovery.

Almost all cancer patients feel overwhelming anxiety, stress, and depression; all of which can impact their immune response. High levels of stress stimulate the production of many hormones and neurotransmitters that reach the tumor microenvironment, as well as activate adrenergic receptors, which can promote tumor progression. At the same time, stress negatively impacts immune cell functioning, making it all the more difficult for the body to fight cancer. For example, in a paper published by Eng, et al. researchers reported that tumors could contain adrenergic receptors, which are associated with increased tumor aggression. Their study also shows that one common biological response to stress is the release of norepinephrine, which is responsible for inhibiting the anti-cancer immune response, while various immune cells, such as Tregs (a type of T cell first discussed in Chapter 2 that helps prevent autoimmune disorders), MDSCs (myeloid-derived suppressor cells), and TAMs (tumor-associated macrophages) may be affected as well, further reducing the immune response. In Eng's, et al. study, mice that were kept at a cooler room temperature, which causes chronic stress, had their tumors grow at a faster rate as compared to the mice kept at a warmer, more comfortable temperature.

This finding suggests that minimizing chronic stress can have a powerful beneficial effect on the immune response.[21] Yet minimizing chronic stress in cancer patients is no easy task. Not only is the cancer diagnosis itself profoundly stressful, but so, too, is the treatment. One area being studied is the effect of chemotherapy treatment on the immune response. There is some evidence that chemotherapy can enhance the immune response; however, there is also concern that it may hurt the immune response. This raises the question "Should immunotherapy be used before chemotherapy?" I think that we will have a better idea of this answer in the next few years, but in the meantime many people are questioning whether prior chemotherapy treatment is hurting the potential for success with immunotherapy treatment. At the moment, it seems certain types of chemotherapy may hurt future success of immunotherapy while others may help it. The book Yoni Keisari has edited, *Tumor Ablation: Effects on Systemic and Local Anti-Tumor Immunity and on Other Tumor Microenvironment Interactions,* has a very good chapter on this subject.

Eng, et al. also cited studies that have shown that stress from surgery results in immune suppression, which inhibits the anti-cancer immune response, increasing the chance of recurrence. Consequently, it is critically important that any treatment plan includes stress-reduction as a fundamental component of therapy.

Toward that end, I've found in my practice that many patients have success with meditation, which helps control the mind and relax the body, and yoga, which works in much the same way as meditation. Having a strong support system is also important, and I encourage my patients' families to be engaged in the treatment plan and understand that they play a vital role in the recovery process.

The impact of surgery on stress levels is another reason that less-invasive procedures such as cryoablation may be a good alternative to conventional surgery when possible. However, when surgery is necessary, it may be possible to counteract some of this effect with Beta blockers, such as the drug Propranolol, which inhibits Beta adrenergic receptors, and thereby helps block stress-induced tumor progression. Clinical studies have indicated that cancer patients using Beta blockers to treat their high blood pressure have improved survival independent from other treatments. One huge advantage is that Beta blockers are already available and can be used off-label.

As these studies and findings show, the immune response and the cancer's ability to evade the immune system create a complex interplay shaped by many different factors. Not only are there different types of cancer, but each cancer can be unique to that patient, with a different immune response irrespective of the cancer type. Also, the same tumor type can have a different immune response based on the tissue it grows in, adding to more complexity.

One thing that is quickly coming of age is our ability to monitor hundreds of immune-related substances in the blood. These advances can allow us to monitor the immune response generated in individual patients, and alter therapies accordingly based on each patient's unique immune response. This certainly will lead to a true personalized medicine and improve treatment outcomes.

One of the most exciting developments in this regard is in computerized data analyses. One such program, IBM's "Watson," has been able to "read" all the studies and findings in cancer research, and make recommendations of treatment options based on a patient's unique biological profile.[22] While access to this computer remains limited, other computerized diagnostic tools are increasingly used by oncologists and other doctors to develop unique treatment profiles. Moreover, because the immune response is so dynamic, continuous monitoring of these immune factors will allow us to adjust treatment and monitor response on the fly, instead of waiting for outcomes of the scans, which can be months down the road.

As I reflect on the successes we have had and on the possibilities before us, I am struck by how rapidly our understanding of cancer and immunotherapy is evolving. There now seems to be an almost limitless number of immune agents being developed and as a result we probably already have a sufficient number of immune agents to cure the majority of cancer patients. And while this vast array of agents adds to the difficulty in fitting the right agent to the right cancer in the right patient, we aren't looking for a single immune agent. Just as we have seen in the treatment of HIV and AIDS, combinations of drugs will be essential to effectively treat cancer. Based on our ongoing work in cancer immunotherapy, we now know that autoimmunity increases when a combination of different agents is used. Moreover, by injecting the agents directly into the tumor, we can help reduce autoimmunity, which makes it easier for the patient to be able to tolerate the combinations needed to have a successful cancer treatment. This is not as possible when given by an IV, flooding the entire body. Some of the necessary drugs like TLR agonist can only be injected into tumors or used topically due to the toxic immune response if used systemically. At this moment, everything in the future of cancer immunotherapy is pointing to having at least some component of intra-tumoral therapy.

This knowledge, combined with the growing number of immune agents, allows for a higher number of combinations of immunotherapies without flooding the body with any one single drug, theoretically reducing the risk of side effects, including autoimmunity. In conventional cancer treatment, the drugs are delivered to the entire body, which can cause debilitating side effects and prove to be more than the patient can tolerate. But by delivering those drugs directly to the tumor, the body is spared the massive dosage of drugs, which instead are focused exclusively on the tumor. Moreover, by directing the drugs to the tumor itself, not only is a lower quantity of the drugs needed, the cost of those drugs is reduced, as well.

As I write these closing lines, I'm encouraged to know that numerous other immune checkpoint agents are close to approval. Among the ones I suspect we will soon see are TIM-3 and LAG-3 which are classified as co-inhibitory receptor targets and are similar to PD-1 and CTLA-4. But unlike those receptors, TIM-3 and LAG-3 have specialized functions at tissue sites.[23]

Another promising area of research is the addition of Toll-Like Receptor Agonist (TLR) with immune checkpoint inhibitors. TLR agonists are a class of proteins that play a key role in the immune system, and when they are directly injected into the tumor, they help activate an immune response that can ultimately translate to specific and long-term immunity. Though TLR is a medication that has been around for years, its use has been limited to a topical cream used to treat genital warts, keratosis, and basal-cell carcinoma. Given new research into the role TLRs play in cancer immunotherapy, however, we are already performing treatments that include injecting TLR agonist CpG, Imiquimod, Resiquimod, and Gardiquimod directly injected into the tumor, combined with cryoablation and immune checkpoint inhibitors. Thus far, the results are extremely promising. Also as mentioned, one of the extremely promising areas of treatment is the injection of an OX40 agonist antibody with a TLR agonist, like in the *Stanford Cancer Vaccine* study published by Levy. We are already working with human patients in this same area as well.

I have found in my work that focusing on the tumor microenvironment is the key to combating cancer. By teaching the immune system to attack the tumor directly, the immune system will go on to attack the cancer in other locations, while not triggering the immune system where no cancer is present. This treatment strategy generates a systemic immune response, also known as an abscopal effect. *Ab* is Latin for "away" and *scopus* is Latin for target, and thus the abscopal effect refers to effects that extend beyond the targeted area. Because of this abscopal effect, it is not necessary to target every tumor in the body to obtain a good response. If there is cancer elsewhere in the body, the immune response can detect it, while the right combination of immunotherapy agents can maximize the anti-cancer response while keeping the immune system from attacking the healthy elements of the body to the lowest possible.[24] This is very important in advanced cancer cases, where it would be almost impossible to target every tumor in the body.

This direct intra-tumoral injection of immunotherapy is my main area of work and is receiving a lot of attention by medical scientists, which is a profound change in cancer care, because it shifts the treatment from oncologists to radiologists. As I've said previously, because oncologists are not trained to perform these procedures and radiologists are, oncologists remain hesitant to refer their patients to radiologists for effective treatment. We therefore need to follow the radical shift in our understanding of cancer treatment, to a radical shift in our paradigm of cancer treatment. As oncologists learn to work alongside radiologists and as radiologists begin to play a more prominent role in cancer treatment, we will completely shake up the cancer world. This is well overdue.

When I began performing ablation on patients in 2002, I started by focusing on breast masses where the cancer had already spread. I was also doing ablations in other parts of the body that were not considered standard at the time, such as bone, lymph nodes, pelvic masses, and adrenal glands. But just as with surgery, we could not get all the cancer, and even if we did, the cancer would usually come back. That is the nature of cancer; there is usually much more cancer in the body than is visible in the scans. It is hiding as microscopic disease, waiting to strike again. That has been the problem with all cancer treatments; rarely can all the cancer be eliminated.

But with immunotherapy injected into the tumor with or without cryoablation that problem is no longer insurmountable. By the end of 2014, with the approval of PD-1 inhibitors Opdivo and Keytruda, we found the key that we'd been missing. That was when we began to see a vaccine-like response, not in one out of every 300 cases as we see with ablation alone, but in a larger number of our patients. The PD-1 inhibitors had opened a door that enabled other agents, once ineffective when used alone, to become far more effective. While the PD-1 inhibitors are not the complete answer and we have a long way to go, they did result in the biggest improvement in patient response that in my view, we have ever before seen in the history of any cancer treatment, at least up until now.

I would argue that while new agents are being developed on a near-daily basis, the agents already exist to make cryoablation combined with immunotherapy an effective cure for cancer in many solid cancers. We've achieved these results with mice, but curing mice is rather easy business; curing humans is what we are after. But the human immune system is far more complex than that of a mouse, which creates added difficulties in treating cancer.

In my own practice, I have developed a combination of approved immune agents, AblationVax™, which I inject into the ablated tumor. The results have been impressive, but we must still refine our procedure if we are going to get to that goal of over 90% success rate. Toward that end, we are studying other agents that have not yet been approved, and I think we are close to reaching our goal. But in order to do so, we need to get these treatments to patients as quickly as possible because time is ticking and people are losing their lives.[25]

Unfortunately, waiting for FDA approval of new but effective agents can take years. In the past few years there have been some major discoveries, but it is frustrating to know that it could take ten to fifteen years for some of these agents to be approved. Dr. Tasuku Honjo of Kyoto University first discovered the immune checkpoint inhibitor PD-1 in 1992, but it wasn't until 2014 that Keytruda, the first PD-1 inhibitor, was approved. While I feel it is critical that we know that the drugs we are using are safe and effective, I can't help but wonder how many people would still be alive today if that drug had come out five years sooner.

Moreover, even when Keytruda was approved, it was approved for melanoma only. Not only did that mean insurance would only cover it for melanoma, it also meant that if a person had another cancer, such as lung or kidney cancer, and asked their doctor for the PD-1 inhibitors, they would inevitably be told, "Oh, that doesn't work for your type of cancer." But approval and effectiveness are not necessarily the same thing. How many patients missed the opportunity to be cured, or at least have their lives extended by years, because their doctor would not step out of the box and offer them immunotherapy?

It is no different with cryoablation and immunotherapy. Patients are typically offered single-agent immunotherapy or cryoablation in place of immunotherapy. But by combining multiple agents with cryoablation, we can save tens of thousands, perhaps even hundreds of thousands, of lives each year. Unfortunately, most doctors want to wait for more studies to prove this treatment strategy will work, ignoring the empirical evidence that already exists demonstrating that this is the way to go. I am confident that the combined treatment of cryoablation with multiple-agent immunotherapy will eventually become accepted as the standard of care. Yet, as I recall watching my grandmother suffer when I was a young teenager, I remember wondering if there was something out there that could help her, something maybe even right under our noses that we just didn't know about. I don't know if it was true back then, but I sure know that it is true now.

Although we can use all approved agents off-label in the U.S., regulations at individual hospitals and insurance limitations have made it virtually impossible to perform our work in the United States. Consequently, my team and I are taking our work outside the U.S. to help speed up this access to new agents for our patients. We have a thriving practice in Mexico City, Mexico but we intend to continue our work in the United States. We currently have an office in Atlanta, Georgia.

I hope that this book has been helpful and has given you some guidance in your cancer care. If you are a doctor who treats cancer patients, I hope I have provided you with enough information to continue researching the topic so that you can better treat and refer your patients. If you are a cancer patient and being treated with immunotherapy, you certainly need to consider the things that can help improve your chance of success, including *Bifido breve* and *longum* and NSAIDS such as Celebrex or aspirin. Clearly, if cryoablation is an option for you, I hope that you will strongly consider that. Cryoablation functions like an immunotherapy on its own, and as you know by now, immunotherapy injected into the tumor at the same time seems to increase the success rate many times more than either on their own. The whole is much greater than the sum of its parts, when it comes to combining cryoablation with multiple-agent immunotherapy.

I do hope that the information you have gained in this book will help you succeed in your battle. I would like to think that my grandmother is looking down and smiling, knowing that her death was not in vain. I am confident that the pieces to the puzzling cure for cancer that we have been searching for are here, right under our noses. This puzzle is quickly coming together, and if you have cancer, your chances for a healthy future have never been greater. I wish you great success.

Frequently Asked Questions

My oncologist doesn't recommend immunotherapy. Should I change oncologists?

Though your oncologist may well have good reasons not to recommend immunotherapy, it would be reasonable to seek a second opinion. It is also important to question your oncologist to get a feel for his or her knowledge of immunotherapy. Because new discoveries regarding immunotherapy are made every day, it's quite possible your doctor isn't aware of all the recent advancements in the field.

How do I find an oncologist who specializes in immuno-therapy?

You can find doctors who use or specialize in immunotherapy on the Society for Immunotherapy of Cancer (SITC) website, www.sitcancer.org

How do I know if I'm a good candidate for immunotherapy?

It's important for patients to take an active role in their own health care and that means that you may need to research a lot of this yourself. Would you trust your cancer care with someone who spends less time with you than your hairdresser? Of course, you wouldn't. But modern healthcare increasingly means you must do just that. Arm yourself with as much information as you can so that you can ask your physician informed questions—and get second and even third opinions if you need to. It's quite possible you are not a good candidate, but it's likely that you are and the more you know about your options, the better decisions you can make regarding your healthcare.

In addition, you may need to seek out doctors who are more open-minded and experienced with immunotherapy, because far too many are reluctant to try treatment strategies they've never employed before.

I can't afford immunotherapy. Should I go ahead and try some of your suggestions anyway, like taking aspirin, probiotics, baking soda and Viagra?

Definitely take *Bifido breve* and l*ongum*, but aspirin, Viagra/ Cialis, and baking soda should only be taken after discussing these with your doctor. Also, I prefer the prescription drug, Protonix to baking soda for affecting the tumor pH, so do ask your doctor if it's a good choice for you. Many of the described medications and supplements may be beneficial, not matter if you are taking immunotherapy, or not.

How do I determine if I am a good candidate for AblationVax™ or intra-tumoral immunotherapy?

At this time there is limited access for patients utilizing these types of treatments. It would be best to have someone experienced in these treatments, such as myself, to review your case and determine if you are a candidate. In general, the best candidates have a solid tumor located in an area that can be accessed with a needle through image guidance. This is actually the majority of patients, as our technology gives us the ability to place needles into tumors in almost every location in the body. Even if patients have failed prior therapy, including immunotherapy, they can still be a good candidate for these procedures.

I'm a woman. Is it safe for me to take my husband's Viagra?

It is safe for women to take Viagra, but you should never take someone else's medicine. Viagra can interact with other drugs and cause reduced blood pressure. Your medical history needs to be evaluated and the medicine needs to be prescribed directly to you by your doctor.

Is immunotherapy safe for children?

Immunotherapy is safe for children and in fact, Yervoy just recently gained approval for pediatric melanoma. I expect we will see more pediatric immunotherapy approvals soon. Many successful clinical trials are being conducted with immunotherapy for children.

Can I schedule a consultation with you?

Yes, you can. Our contact information is on our website at www.WilliamsCancerInstitute.com. Our clinic sites are rapidly growing and I consult with patients both in the U.S. and in several Latin American countries.

What are the side effects of immunotherapy?

Immunotherapy often results in fatigue while your body is fighting the cancer. This fatigue can last a few weeks to a few months. The other issue with immunotherapy is that it can create autoimmune problems. Skin rash is the most common, which usually responds well to topical steroid cream. Autoimmune reactions are seen in many locations, including the thyroid, lung, and liver. These reactions can be also treated with steroids, and studies suggest that using steroids does not reduce the effectiveness of immunotherapy. It is very important, however, that you are monitored closely and that your doctor understands these risks, so that if a problem develops you are treated promptly.

Besides your doctor monitoring labs for liver and thyroid problems, any shortness of breath needs to be reported to your doctor immediately to rule out autoimmune inflammation of the lung (autoimmune pneumonitis). This is a rare occurrence, but a more serious issue that needs to be treated. It may sound a little scary, but in general patients do well and are far happier with immunotherapy than other cancer treatments. Also I might add that immunotherapy is not associated with some of the toxic side effects often seen with chemotherapy, like hair loss.

I have leukemia. Can immunotherapy help me?

When it comes to blood cancers, such as leukemia, there are immunotherapy treatments using engineered T cells (called Car-T). There are some that were recently approved.

What should I look for when choosing an oncologist or another cancer specialist?

For a cancer patient it is most important that you take control of your care and don't just follow recommendations blindly. Do your own research. When a doctor suggests a treatment, really question what are the potential results. Most patients are shocked to find in many cases of advanced cancer, that treatments such as chemotherapy may only offer a few months increase in survival. Keep in mind that a doctor is only thinking about your case the few minutes you see them. It is not their fault; it is the system that requires high volumes of patients. There is just no time for a doctor to dedicate extensive time to any one case. There are constantly new developments that doctors will not be aware of. As for the doctor, you want someone open-minded enough to listen to the suggestions you have come up with from good research. Certainly you need to look for information that is based on good science, there is a lot of information out there, but there needs to be real science to support it. Your doctor must be open-minded to supplements and off-label medications. They should realize that just because they do not know or understand a treatment, it does not mean that it is useless. They should be willing to look at the data and give different ideas a genuine consideration. When you meet your doctor, bring a very concise list of ideas that you have come up with, or even bring this book. I would not just overwhelm them with a giant stack of research papers. If there is something that you feel really strong about, bring a few of the abstracts or summaries. Keep in mind that they only have minutes to deal with your case, so too much info is probably going to just be ignored. If the doctor responds positively, then you may have someone you can work with. If not, you may want to keep looking. The only way the oncologist will get the

THE IMMUNOTHERAPY REVOLUTION

message and hopefully become more receptive is that you have to vote with your feet.

Where can I find more information about immunotherapy?

I have posted additional information on my website and blog www.WilliamsCancerInstitute.com. For the most up-to-date information, you can follow me on:

Twitter: @jasonwilliamsmd

Instagram: @immunotherapyforcancer and @immunotherapy_revolution_book

Facebook: @cryoimmunotherapy

Soon we will be hosting a podcast. The Society for Immunotherapy of Cancer (SITC) website, www.sitcancer.org is also an excellent source for information.

Resources

Oncology Nursing Society hosts an immunotherapy discussion group: www.communities.ons.org/communities/community-home?CommunityKey=dc258d3d-a23d-41a6-8799-5c9f1dbbbe27

The Immunotherapy Foundation is a nonprofit organization that funds immunotherapy research. They post updates on the most recent research: www.TheImmunoTherapyFoundation.org/news-and-resources

CancerCare provides counseling, support and financial aid to cancer patients, and here is a link to their podcasts about immunotherapy: www.cancercare.org/tagged/immunotherapy

The Society for Immunotherapy of Cancer (SITC) website is, as I've said previously, an excellent resource: www.sitcancer.org.

For more in-depth reading on tumor ablation, Yoni Keisari has edited a very good book, *Tumor Ablation: Effects on*

Systemic and Local Anti-Tumor Immunity and on Other Tumor Microenvironment Interactions (Springer Publications, 2013). At $169 for an e-book, it might be beyond the budget of most people, but I especially recommend it for oncologists: www. springer.com/us/book/9789400746930

Acknowledgements

THERE ARE MANY people that I would like to thank who have helped make my career and this book possible. First and foremost, I thank my parents, Jim and Lois. Unfortunately, my father passed away during the writing of this book, but he was still able to give me great guidance that I believe sent this book in a better direction. My mother Lois has always been the best mother a son could ever ask for. It has been the love and support and unending belief in me that my parents provided which have allowed me to become the person I am today.

To my children, Ryan, Blake and Caroline. I thank you for your sacrifice and understanding of how this war against cancer has taken much of my time away from you guys. I hope that this work will make you proud. I am certainly proud of each of you.

To my wife, Stefanya. You are the love of my life and best friend. I thank you for your unconditional love and support and for bringing joy to my life while I continue this quest to rid the world of this dreadful disease. It would be a long and lonely road without you.

To Angie Holder and Ashley Willis. Thank you for always sticking by my side. You have become my extended family. This work would not be possible without your help and support.

To my friend and colleague, Dr. Mark Rosenberg. Thank you for our long discussions into cancer treatments and believing in my work.

To Dr. Carlos Vargas and Eduardo Cortes. Thank you for all that you do in helping provide the best care for patients.

To my friend and colleague, Dr. Dwight McKee. Thank you for sharing your wisdom with me over all these years which has been instrumental in guiding me in the right path.

To my good friend, Rob Risman. Thank you for always having faith in me and for being a good friend. I want to thank you and your family for the support of our research at Case Western Reserve University.

To Dr. Alex Haung of Case Western Reserve University. Thank you for being excited about this work and willing to join me to study this further for the advancement of patient care.

To the researchers from the Society for Immunotherapy of Cancer (SITC), this work literally comes from me standing on the shoulders of giants. It is your work in the trenches of the labs that has made you the true heroes in cancer research.

To Dr. Patrick Sewell. Thank you for your early innovation and pioneering ideas in ablation which helped shape the direction my career has taken. I always value our continued work together and friendship.

To Claudia Salerno. Thank you for all your hard work and dedication in the assistance of publishing this book. Your vision and ideas are "a breath of fresh air."

I wish to thank my grandmother, Effie Jenkins McIntyre, to whom this book is dedicated. I see you in each of my patients. You are continually in my thoughts and you are my motivation to continue in my cancer research. I know it is far too late for you, but I feel that you are very proud of all I have done to save others from this tragic disease.

Finally, to my patients, past, present and future. I have learned so much from you. It is for you that I do what I do. I hope that no more will a family have to suffer the loss of a loved one due to this dreaded disease. I wish you a long happy life, cancer-free.

About the Author

D R. JASON R. WILLIAMS is a medical doctor, board-certified radiologist, image-guided cancer specialist, researcher, and professor. He is one of the pioneers of immunotherapy, specializing in intra-tumoral interventions. He performed the world's first ablation procedure and implemented an intra-tumoral injection of a specific combination of immunotherapy agents, thus leveraging the actual process of ablation as an immunotherapy agent itself. Since then, he has performed thousands of procedures—many of them "first in human"—in multiple areas of ablation and cryoablation therapies.

Dr. Williams is the Director of Interventional Oncology and Immunotherapy at the Williams Cancer Institute, where he has been advancing the use of intra-tumoral immunotherapy. He is also an adjunct professor at Case Western Reserve University in Cleveland, Ohio, where he is helping to further cutting-edge research. In addition, he is actively involved in private research combining numerous different immunotherapy agents for image-guided intra-tumoral injection covering almost all cancer types. He lives part-time in Atlanta, Georgia and Mexico City, Mexico. To learn more about Dr. Williams and his clinic, visit www.WilliamsCancerInstitute.com.

Committed to further advance research in intra-tumoral immunotherapy and help those who are struggling financially to cover medical care, Dr. Williams is donating all proceeds from this book for this cause.

***

If you are interested in purchasing this book in bulk, please contact us directly through our websites:

www.ImmunotherapyRevolution.com
www.WilliamsCancerInstitute.com

Endnotes

1   https://www.cancer.gov/about-cancer/understanding/
    statistics

2   Den Brok, Martijn H.M.G.M., et al. (2006) "Synergy
    between *in situ* cryoblation and TLRN stimulation
    results in a highly effective *In vivo* dendritic cell vaccine,"
    Cancer Research 66:14:7285-7292.

3   Marabelle, Aurélien, Holbrook Kohrt, and Ronald Levy,
    (2013)Department of Medicine, Division of Oncology,
    Stanford University, "Intratumoral Anti-CTLA-4 Ther-
    apy: Enhancing Efficacy While Avoiding Toxicity,"*Clin
    Cancer Res.* 19(19): October 1. doi:10.1158/1078-0432.
    CCR-13-1923.

4   Ibid.

5   Vétizou, Marie, et al. (2015) "Anti-cancer immunother-
    apy by CTLA-4 blockade relies on the gut microbiota,"
    Science 350:6264:1079-1084, November 27.

6   Kubo, Isao, et al. (1993) "Antitumor agents from the
    cashew (*Anacardiumoccidentale*) apple juice," *Journal of
    Agricultural and Food Chemistry,* 41(6):1012-1015.

7   Hollands, Andrew, et al. (2016) "Natural Product Anacardic Acid from Cashew Nut Shells Stimulates Neutrophil Extracellular Trap Production and Bactericidal Activity," Journal of Biological Chemistry, available online at: http://www.jbc.org/cgi/doi/10.1074/jbc.M115.695866

8   Frankel, Arthur E., et al. (2017) "Metagenomic Shotgun Sequencing to identify specific human gut microbes associated with immune checkpoint therapy efficacy in melanoma patients," Poster presentation at the *American Society of Clinical Oncology*, Chicago, Illinois, June 3. Forthcoming in *J Clin Oncol* 35, 2017.

9   Hawk ET, Viner JL, Umar A, *et al.* (2003) "Cancer and the cyclooxygenase enzyme: Implications for treatment and prevention," *Am J Cancer* 2003; 2:27–55.

10 Nakanishi, Y., et al. (2011) "COX-2 inhibition alters the phenotype of tumor-associated macrophages from M2 to M1 in ApcMin/1 mouse polyps," *Carcinogenesis* 32:9:1333–1339.

11 Hennequart, M., et al. (2017) Constitutive IDO1 expression in human tumors is driven by cyclooxygenase-2 and mediates intrinsic immune resistance. *Cancer Immunology Research* DOI: 10.1158/2326-6066.CIR-16-0400 (2017); *Science Daily* press release.

12 Yi, Yongkui, et al. (2016) *Oncoimmunology* 5:2: e1074374-4.

13 Forget, P., et al. (2014) "Intraoperative use of ketorolac or diclofenac is associated with improved disease-free survival and overall survival in conservative breast cancer surgery," *British Journal of Anaesthesia* 113(S1): i82–i87.

14 Nakanishi, Y., et al. (2011) "COX-2 inhibition alters the phenotype of tumor-associated macrophages from M2 to M1 in ApcMin/1 mouse polyps," *Carcinogenesis* 32:9:1333–1339.

15 Weatherall, M. W., et al. (2010) "Intravenous aspirin (lysine acetylsalicylate) in the inpatient management of headache,"*American Academy of Neurology*, 75:12:1098-1103.

16 Barreira da Silva, et al. (2015) "Dipeptidylpeptidase 4 inhibition enhances lymphocyte trafficking, improving both naturally occurring tumor immunity and immunotherapy," *Nature Immunology*, 16:850-858.

17 Serafini, Paolo, et al. (2006) JEM © The Rockefeller University Press 203:12: 2691–2702, November 27. www.jem.org/cgi/doi/10.1084/jem.20061104.

18 Brand, A., et al. (2016) *Cell Metabolism* 24:657–671, November 8, 2016. Elsevier Inc.

19 Pilon-Thomas, S., et al. (2015) "Neutralization of Tumor Acidity Improves Antitumor Responses to Immunotherapy," *Cancer Research*; 76:6:1381-1390, March 15, 2016.

20 Vishvakarma, N. (2010) "Immunopotentiating effect of proton pump inhibitor Pantoprazole in a lymphoma-bearing murine host: implication in antitumor activation of tumor-associated macrophages," *Immunology Letters* 134:83-92.

21 Eng, Jason W., et al. (2014) "A Nervous Tumor Microenvironment: The Impact of Adrenergic Stress on Cancer Cells, Immunosuppression, and Immunotherapeutic Response," *Cancer ImmunolImmunother*.2014 November 63(11): 1115–1128.

22 https://www.mskcc.org/about/innovative-collabora
    tions/watson-oncology

23 Anderson, A.C., N. Joller and V.K. Kuchroo (2016)
    "Lag-3, Tim-3, and TIGIT: Co-inhibitory Receptors
    with Specialized Functions in Immune Regulation,"
    Immunity, 2016 May 17;44(5):989-1004. doi: 10.1016/j.
    immuni.2016.05.001.

24 Cross, Ryan. c&en, Vol 96 Issue 9 pp. 24-26, Feb 26,
    2018; "STING fever is sweeping through the cancer
    immunotherapy world."

25 Wang, et al. Front Pharmacolgy, 2018, Mar 5; "Com-
    bining Immunotherapy and Radiotherapy for Cancer
    Treatment: Current Challenges and Future Directions."